D1606328

With Stethoscope and Scapular

With Stethoscope and Scapular

by Joseph C. Evers, M. D.

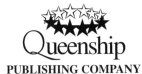

Queenship
PUBLISHING COMPANY
P.O Box 42028 Santa Barbara, CA 93140-2028
(800) 647-9882 • (805) 957-4893 • Fax: (805) 957-1631

Dedication

1. To God's Infinite Mercy gifted to us all through Jesus Christ's redemptive sacrifice on Calvary's hill.
2. To Mary Immaculate, the Mother of God and our spiritual mother.
3. To Mary Ann and Cathy.
4. To my wife Jean, our children Joe, Sharon, Tara and Lisa, their spouses Barbara, Larry and Rob, our good friend Mike and our grandchildren, Taylor, Ryan, Colbert, Jordan Elizabeth and Cristen Anne.

Cover photo: © L'Osservatore Romano, used with permission.

©1996 Queenship Publishing

Library of Congress Number # 96-67917

Published by:
Queenship Publishing
P.O. Box 42028
Santa Barbara, CA 93140-2028
(800) 647-9882 • (805) 957-4893 • Fax: (805) 957-1631

Printed in the United States of America

ISBN: 1-882972-70-8

Contents

Acknowledgments

I would like to express my sincere thanks to Helen De Hart who first read and edited the manuscript. Without her enthusiasm and help on the text, I doubt that this book would have ever materialized. Also, I would like to thank Pat Canes who offered many helpful suggestions when I was first seeking a publisher. Finally, and in a particular manner I would like to thank Mrs. Carol Wilcox of Tan Publishers. The book was in moth balls for a number of years when Carol read it and encouragingly said "This book must find a publisher." She, an editor by profession, help me to polish up the manuscript and to find a publisher.

— 1 —

An Easter Story

An event occurred in my life many years ago involving one of God's young children that provided me with an instantaneous glimpse into the unfathomable depths of God's love and mercy. Easter was but a week away, and I was just completing my second-year residency training in pediatrics at Metropolitan Children's Hospital. The cold, dreary days of winter were but an unpleasant memory as soft spring sunshine bathed the metropolitan area. I had been working all morning in the outpatient department, drawing blood samples from young children. It was all part of a viral research project with the virology team at the hospital. An attractive young nurse by the name of Jean had been helping me. I noticed how gentle and caring she was with the children — and yet at the same time, how she was so very efficient. I made a silent resolution to ask her out on a date sometime in the near future.

After completing the work in the outpatient department, I went upstairs to the third-floor rooftop outdoor enclosure for a breath of fresh air and surveyed the city below. Tulips and daffodils dotted occasional small, green lawns, giving a modicum of life to the maze of sidewalks and streets.

The outpatient therapy unit for crippled children abutted the outdoor enclosure, and as I breathed in the sights and odors of the morning, the joyous notes of children's laughter rippled through the air as young, smiling student nurses laughed and played with them.

The hospital census was light, and I had finished rounds early on my assigned infectious disease unit and was enjoying this pleasant interlude when the hospital intercom announced, "Adolescent rounds on Fifth Floor Main commencing in five minutes; adolescent rounds on Fifth Floor Main commencing in five minutes."

The new head of the Adolescent Department had recently joined the staff, and with time on my hands and feeling a tinge of guilt over my outdoor escape, I decided I might as well accompany the students and residents on teaching rounds and gather whatever pearls of wisdom the new Chief might offer.

Within minutes I joined the group, and with the Chief in the lead, about nine or ten of us entered an eight-bed ward containing young adolescent males ranging from thirteen to eighteen years of age.

We clustered about the first bed, in which lay a sixteen-year-old boy with a confusing diagnostic problem. His long history demanded a lengthy, detailed presentation by the third-year medical student, and as he droned on with the intricacies of the case I found myself impatiently shifting from foot to foot, visually surveying the large eight-bed room. That's when I first became aware of him.

A young boy, very seriously ill, was sitting on the edge of the bed, his body drenched with perspiration, struggling for air with every breath. The palpitations of his heart, fully visible, were erratically tapping a macabre dance on his chest wall. The whites of his eyes, stained a deep yellow, met mine and silently pleaded for help.

The group eventually reached the boy. His name was John; he was thirteen. He had metastatic carcinoma, and it had invaded all of his abdominal organs. His liver, completely filled with tumor cells, was no longer functioning, and its failure was responsible for the generalized jaundiced hue of his skin and for the large accumulation of fluid which completely filled his abdominal cavity. He was in the terminal stages of the disease.

Now only a few feet away from me, he was a pitiful sight. The taut, parchment-like yellow skin covering his bloated abdomen looked as though it would burst at any moment. He looked so helpless, so much in agony and so abandoned... I felt grief-stricken realizing that all medical avenues to cure his illness or even to alleviate his suffering had been exhausted.

Rounds eventually ended, and despondently I left the ward and went to the nurses' station. Out of curiosity, I reviewed his chart. It was most depressing. His hospital stay had been lengthy, visitations from immediate family and other relatives few, and his disease had relentlessly progressed with a vengeance, gradually weakening him physically and mentally.

I glanced at the section indicating religious denomination. My heart sank, for boldly printed in he small designated, outlined area was the word, "None."

Returning to my duties, I was haunted by the boy's tortured face and grotesquely distorted body. I could not escape the strong urge to do something, anything, to let him know that someone loved him — that someone cared.

I was in the cafeteria eating lunch with four other residents as the next hour passed by swiftly. Turning to the resident responsible for the Adolescent Unit, I asked, "How long has the boy with terminal cancer in the eight-bed ward been ill?"

"I don't know; I think he has been there about a month."

"Has he ever had any visitors?"

"I haven't seen any."

I sadly shook my head and responded, "That's terrible! He seems so alone."

The conversation drifted to other matters, and I continued to eat my lunch silently. Suddenly and unexpectedly an overpowering urge took possession of me to return to 5 Main. Not waiting to finish lunch and not knowing exactly why, I excused myself and hurried to the elevator.

As the elevator inched its way to the fifth floor, my heart started pounding. What if I was too late? The boy looked so ill just a scant two hours ago.

The elevator finally stopped, having completed its laborious climb to 5 Main. I departed and ran down the corridor, sidestepping several personnel approaching in the opposite direction. Careening around the corner, I entered the eight-bed ward.

"Thank God," I sighed; he was still alive. His arms dangled limply over the side-bar of the bed, his head resting on them. His chest cavity moved with great effort, attempting to somehow satisfy the hunger of his air-starved lungs. His lips were blue as beads of perspiration pock-marked his face and saliva dribbled from the corner of his mouth. His eyes met mine and seemed to be saying, "Please, please, help me."

The thought of baptizing the boy impulsively occurred to me. The glories of the Sacrament raced through my mind: complete remission of sin, not only Original Sin, but even the temporal punishment due to actual sin. Even more glorious, instantaneous admission into the family of God.

Some gauze absorbent pads were near the washbasin. I quickly grasped them and saturated them with water as I approached the bed. "John, have you ever heard of Jesus?"

He painfully nodded his head.

"He is God's Son, and He died for us on the Cross so we could live with Jesus forever. Would you like to live with Jesus forever, John?"

Once again, he weakly moved his head up and down.

Squeezing the water over his head and forehead, I solemnly pronounced the words, "I baptize you in the name of the Father, and of the Son, and of the Holy Ghost. Amen."

As soon as I had finished, I embraced him. John looked up into my eyes, and with a slight but unmistakable smile, breathed his last and died. Gazing at him, now looking so peaceful, I recalled St. Paul's words: "The eye has not seen, nor the ear heard, nor has it entered into the hearts of man the joys that God has prepared for those who love Him."

— 2 —

The Promise of Eternity

The Fatima apparitions of the Blessed Mother and her urgent requests delivered to three small Portuguese children had long held my fascination. It was inconceivable to me that the three innocent seers of Fatima could have fabricated or imagined the events. After all, had not all Pontiffs within recent memory given the apparitions of Our Lady their blessings?

It was an unusual avocation for a pediatric chief resident, but totally convinced of their authenticity and urgency, I had joined forces with a small band of like-minded persons and started touring different Catholic parishes. I would talk to interested groups numbering from twenty to as many as one hundred or more, reiterating the Blessed Mother's plea for the daily Rosary, penance, and sacrifice. I had been dating Jean for awhile now, and on occasion she would accompany me to these presentations. Particularly emphasized at each presentation was the importance of consecrating oneself to the Immaculate heart of Mary and of wearing the Brown Scapular. At each talk's conclusion, I would hold up a scapular for all to see and recall its heavenly promise: "Whosoever dies wearing this scapular shall not suffer eternal fire."

I had long ago formed the Fatima habit of a personal daily Rosary, and for its recitation I frequently went to a neighboring hospital chapel dedicated to the Immaculate heart of Mary. In addition, I had made it a practice to make a novena to Our Lady of Fatima once or twice a year. In fact, it was on May 5, the first day of my novena to Our Lady of Fatima, at Sacred Heart Church, that I proposed to Jean and placed her engagement ring on her finger.

Since that beautiful moment, our love has never wavered for one another and has truly deepened throughout the years. I thank God for our life together.

It was in the early spring that I first met Bill while praying my Fatima Rosary in Our Lady's chapel. The soft glow of reflected candlelight revealed his firm yet gentle features, which radiated love as he stood with eyes gazed upward at the beautiful Madonna statue that was placed to the right of the altar.

His lean, muscular body was clothed in the traditional whites of a fourth-year medical student. A clipboard was tucked under his left arm. For what seemed an endless moment, he seemed transfixed before the statue of the Virgin: then suddenly, breaking the magnetism, he reverently genuflected before the main altar and exited from the chapel.

Almost simultaneously, I left and in the small foyer outside the chapel door, he looked at me with boyish innocence and exclaimed, "Isn't she wonderful?" Extending his hand, he introduced himself.

"Hi, my name's Bill McCarthy." His grip had strength and character.

"Nice to meet you, Bill; my name is Dr. Joe Evers. Do you come here often?"

"No, not really; I usually go to the chapel in the medical school or to my parish church, Our Lady of Victory, nearby."

"Oh!" I answered, "that explains why I haven't seen you."

"Yeah, I find it more convenient to do that, but I must say, I really like this chapel."

"I know what you mean, Bill; I feel the same way. I couldn't help but notice you admiring the statue of the Blessed Mother; you must be very devoted to her."

His eyes sparkled as he replied, "I am, Doctor; she has been in my corner for as long as I can remember."

"I feel the same way, Bill. Say, if you're interested, I will be giving a talk on the Fatima apparitions in your own parish, Our Lady of Victory, early in May. Why not come?"

"Sounds great, Doctor; you'll probably see me."

The warm feeling of my chance encounter with this young man lingered with me long after our parting.

I savored with each breath the odors of the perfume-laden evening as I motored up the twisting driveway to Our Lady of Victory church.

I began the talk at 8:00 PM and found it well received by the fifty or
so people assembled. They seemed genuinely interested in the
Blessed Mother's Fatima requests, and judging from the questions
that followed, they were eager to put them into practice.

While leaving the church, I was startled by the sudden appearance of Bill McCarthy. For some reason, I had failed to recognize
him in the audience.

"Dr. Evers, I enjoyed your talk."

"Thanks, Bill; glad you could make it."

With a quizzical look, he continued. "For some reason which I
can't quite understand, this is the first time I've ever heard about
the Brown Scapular and its promise. It's fantastic. Why don't people
talk about it more?"

"I wish I could answer that one, Bill, but it's a mystery to me.
Here, I have an extra one." Digging into my pocket, I offered it to
him. "Take it."

His face reflected the joy of a child opening his big present on
Christmas day.

"Gee, thanks, Doctor." He held it in his hands, looking at it.
"Thank you so very much."

"You're welcome, Bill. By the way, it's blessed."

"One more moment of your time, Doctor. You mentioned
something in your talk about being properly enrolled. How do I
go about it?"

"Easy! Any priest can enroll you. In fact, if you are planning to
go to Confession this Saturday, why not have the priest enroll you
after he finishes hearing your confession."

"Great idea; that's just what I will do."

We continued talking for awhile, and I recall how he kept thanking me for this new spiritual discovery. As we departed, I remember what a pleasant glow I experienced, knowing I had played a
small but important role in clothing the Blessed Mother's spiritual
child, Bill, in her livery.

It was three weeks later when I was making pediatric rounds at
the hospital that I recognized Bill's medical student roommate. I
hailed him and inquired how he and Bill were doing. He looked at
me thunderstruck as I spoke.

"You must not have heard; Bill drowned in a canoeing accident on the river three weeks ago."

7

I was speechless as he related the tragic news and continued the sad narrative.

"I remember how happy he was the evening before he died. He had been to Confession that afternoon, and the priest had enrolled him in the scapular that you had given him. He was overjoyed. The very next day, he died."

Tears of sorrow welled up in my eyes for my departed friend, but they were soon replaced by tears of joy as I reflected on the Blessed Mother's promise. I felt secure in the knowledge that Bill was now eternally happy with our Creator and his "wonderful" Madonna.

— 3 —

Jean

With her raven black hair and large, magnetic eyes, she was as beautiful a bride as any budding pediatrician ever could have hoped to call his own. Jean and I were married in Sacred Heart Church on July 16, the Feast of Our Lady of Mount Carmel. Fanned by a gentle breeze, with fluffy white clouds dotting a deep blue sky, the day was as perfect as any bridal couple could wish for.

Prior to our marriage, I had been in solo practice for a year, renting a small, one-floor white painted brick house which I had converted into an office. It had a good location on a busy thoroughfare and it was to this castle, following a five-day honeymoon, that I carried my bride.

It was a cleverly camouflaged castle. During office hours the living room served as a waiting room, while the bedrooms, now unrecognizable as such, made perfect examination rooms. The kitchen masqueraded as a medical laboratory. At 7:00 AM sharp the tablecloth and salt and pepper shakers were removed from the breakfast table and a microscope, microscope lamp and blood counting chamber were substituted. The oven, with the thermostat set on warm, served as a perfect incubator for throat cultures. The polio vaccine was safely tucked in the freezer section of the refrigerator among our frozen foods and ice cubes. The diphtheria, tetanus and pertussis injectables and sterile culture plates nestled comfortable alongside the eggs and bacon. Jean used to tease me now and then with the remark, "Don't be surprised if someday your iced tea is laced with polio vaccine, Sweetheart."

Our bedroom, once a dining room, was separated from the office waiting room by a folding, louvered door which afforded little privacy or protection from disease. Every cough and sneeze floated through the slats in the door into the bedroom. Jean frequently would ask me, "Isn't there something we can disinfect this place with, Darling? And don't be funny and say 'Use a fly swatter.'"

Oh, yes, I forgot to mention that our only bathroom was a public facility during office hours.

Two months after our wedding, Jean was pregnant. She developed morning sickness — what a dreadful affliction. All the anti-nauseates known to medical science failed to help Jean. We used to keep a bucket by the bed in case she couldn't make it to the bathroom, or in case it was already occupied by one of my patients.

"Why do they call it morning sickness, Darling?" she used to ask me sadly. "I'm sick all day and all night."

There were occasions when the nausea left, and then these strange cravings would take possession of her. One of them was exceptionally weird. In fact, nowhere could I find a report of it in the medical literature. She loved the smell of automobile exhaust fumes. A real treat for her was for both of us to be stalled in traffic with the car window open. She would say with genuine satisfaction, "Doesn't that smell divine, Sweetheart?"

"Honey," I would reply, "it actually smells awful. How can you stand it?"

"Oh, it smells so good."

I've often wondered since whether all that carbon monoxide she sucked into her lungs might have been the stumbling block toward our eldest and only son from becoming another Einstein. It could not have affected him too much, however, since he is a physician now.

At 1:00 AM, Jean's nausea completely gone but replaced by a ravenous hunger, the steak and cheese mania would strike her. Not just ANY steak and cheese, mind you, but only one piled high with onions and smothered in mustard. Only such a delicacy from a particular all-night carryout fifteen miles away in the inner city would satisfy her appetite.

The routine became predictable. Awakening from my sleep, I sensed her tossing and turning. Then, with both of us awake, she would gently tap me on the shoulder and sweetly coo, "Aren't you hungry, Dear?"

"No, not again," I would groan.

"I'm starving, and the fresh air will be good for us..." Then, knowing I would not refuse, she would say, "Let's go, Joseph."

Minutes later we would be chugging toward the city, window open, with my good wife leaning to inhale whatever traces of auto exhaust were there for the offering. A weary hour later, her addiction and hunger satisfied, we would return to our love nest and stumble back into bed.

I used to harbor some worrisome thoughts of what the neighbors and townsfolk might be whispering.

"Why yes, the poor dear is losing more and more weight every time I see her."

"And she looks so pale."

"He carries her out in the wee hours of the night, don't you know, and heads toward the city."

"Half out the window she is, they say. Trying to escape, I suppose."

Such thoughts, I'm sure, were nothing more than the product of a young pediatrician's imagination. However, one evening an incident did occur.

For about five days I had been treating Valencia Van Allen (just turned 13 years old) with fluids and anti-fever medication. She had had a fever during this period of time, and I did not know the cause of it.

Mrs. Van Allen called me early one evening, extremely anxious about her daughter.

"Dr. Evers, Valencia is running a temperature of 103 degrees and she not only feels terrible, but looks absolutely horrid as well. Please, can't you do something?"

There was a note of exasperation in her voice, and I had the distinct impression that she was fed up with the new, young doctor in town telling her not to worry and that the fever would soon pass. I had seen the child and had been convinced it was a harmless virus. Now, however, I was starting to feel a bit anxious myself; after all, the poor kid had been ill for five days, and in her mother's eyes I had done little in the way of diagnosis or treatment.

"Mrs. Van Allen, bring Valencia over to the office right now. The door is unlatched, so come right in."

I was doing some paperwork in one of the examining rooms, which also served as a consultation room, when I heard them enter.

Jean, feeling a little worse than usual, was trying to sleep in the bedroom.

I heard the Van Allens enter. Swinging the consultation room door open, I greeted them, "Hi, how are you doing?"

"Not very well, Dr. Evers...just look at her."

Valencia, a little flushed, did not look desperately ill. I explained to them that I was in the midst of some paperwork and asked if they would mind waiting a bit. There was no objection, so I closed the door and returned to my desk.

I despise paperwork. I'd rather crawl bare-kneed and bear-knuckled over red-hot coals than wade through the endless mounds of insurance forms, correspondence and fourth-class mail that makes me forget what the top of my desk look like. But once started on it, I hate interrupting the momentum.

It was for this reason that I kept them waiting a little longer than usual. The door to the consultation room was thick and well-made, and performing well its function of deadening sounds originating from the waiting room. So it was with some surprise and curiosity that I heard through the door intermittent strange muffled noises spaced by indecipherable mumbling from Valencia and her mother. After some ten minutes of this, I could tolerate the suspense no longer. Opening the door a crack, I peeked out and immediately spied the two of them, Valencia kneeling, her mother standing, with their ears next to the white louvered door.

As I opened the door wider so that I was fully visible, Mrs. Van Allen saw me and shrieked, "Oh, Dr. Evers, I'm so glad to see you. I know Valencia is ill, but your poor dog must be twice as ill. She keeps retching and gasping for air."

"Yikes," I thought to myself, "Jean was having another bout of morning sickness and they thought it was a sick pet." Rather than try to explain, I quickly showed them into an examining room, excused myself, and skipped through the kitchen into the bedroom. Jean, by the time I had reached her, had managed to crawl from the bucket she had been using and back into bed.

Glaring at me, she angrily whispered, "What took you so long, didn't you hear me? Those patients of yours thought I was an animal." She was so weak that she had to catch her breath before getting out the next sentence.

"Do you know what they kept asking me through that door? 'What's you name, little doggy? Fido? Spot?' Then the girl squeaked, 'Poor, sick little doggy. Probably choking on a bone.'" With an exasperated sigh Jean added, "If I wasn't so sick I would have growled."

Masking a smile as best as I could, I tucked her in, offered her something to stop the nausea and begged her forgiveness for not having come sooner. She grunted a few times as I patted her hand gently, kissed her on the forehead and returned to my patient.

Determined to ignore any questions relative to my sick "doggy," I entered the examining room and found Valencia lying down on the examining table.

In a rather demanding tone I said, "Valencia, it can't be that bad. Sit up and let me have a look at you."

Spiritlessly, she struggled to a sitting position. Before either of them could utter a word, I asked Valencia to say "Ah." The odor was overpowering. Her tonsils were loaded with pus and four times the normal size. I inquired whether she had any new symptoms.

"Yes, Doctor, she has developed some lumps in her neck and says her throat hurts more."

"I'm not surprised about the throat. Her tonsils are full of infection and look terrible."

Valencia winced as I palpated her cervical lymph nodes. They were very enlarged, and she was in obvious pain and justifiably feeling horrible.

The abdominal exam, I thought to myself, would be important. "Why don't you lie down, Valencia?"

Reluctantly she obliged. I had a suspicion of what I would find. Palpating her abdomen very carefully, I was not surprised to find her spleen swollen and measuring four fingers' breadths below the margin of the left rib cage.

"Mrs. Van Allen, your daughter's spleen is enlarged."

"What does it all mean, Doctor?"

"Valencia has infectious mononucleosis, a rather common disease of young teenagers. Tomorrow I will order some blood tests to confirm my suspicion. If that is what she has, I must warn you she's going to be in bed for the next week and probably home from school for two or three weeks."

Mrs. Van Allen looked momentarily stunned, then replied, "Infectious mononucleosis, how awful." Putting her arms around her daughter affectionately and hugging her she added, "You poor dear, but at least we know what's wrong with you."

Then slowly turning toward me, she condescendingly asked, "And how's that poor doggy?"

I felt like screaming, "Forget my poor doggy!" Some of the parents of my patients had not known about my recent marriage, and the Van Allens obviously were among this group.

Deliberate lying I cannot do, so hoping against hope they wouldn't hear me, I limply replied in a barely audible voice, "I don't have a doggy, Mrs. Van Allen, that's my — — my — wife."

Speechless, Mrs. Van Allen started nervously twisting her handkerchief while her daughter, bewildered, starting whispering as though I were unable to hear her. "Mama, did — he — say — his, his — wife?"

"Dr. Evers," Mrs. Van Allen's voice assumed a rapid, nervous hum, "you did say your wife, you did, didn't you?"

"Yes, I did, Mrs. Van Allen, we were married about three months ago and I'm afraid she has a touch of morning sickness."

Mrs. Van Allen, now calmer, blushed as she responded, "Oh, the poor dear, and to think we thought it was your doggy." Pausing, searching for the right phrase, she continued, "Please ask her to forgive us."

Following a reflective silence she added, "You should really be attending her, Doctor. That morning sickness can be so dreadful!"

"Yes, I know, but she's feeling much better now."

Still feeling uncomfortable over the incident and wishing they would leave, I gave the mother more instructions concerning Valencia and escorted them toward the door. Following a few more embarrassed and embarrassing smiles, they finally left.

The next time I saw Valencia, which was but a few days later, she presented me with an unusually shaped wrapped gift.

She said, "Dr. Evers, would you please give this to Mrs. Evers? It's a bottle of lemon juice with sugar...it always makes me feel better when I get sick to my stomach."

Years later I was to come across a book entitled, Mes*sage of Merciful Love to Little Souls*. It consists of a series of dialogues between Jesus and a chosen soul by the name of Marguerite. The book carries an Imprimatur and a Nihil obstat and attracts a wide audience. It has a spiritual likeness to St. Therese of Lisieux' "Little Way of Spiritual Childhood."

I recall reading the words of Jesus to Marguerite concerning those who aspire to Spiritual Childhood. He says:

> For the Order of Little Souls:
> a sole Master, God;
> a sole guide, My Mother;
> a little instrument, you:
> a single way: abandonment within My arms.
> First enemy to conquer: your ego.
> First virtue to acquire: generosity.

I wonder if Mrs. Van Allen realized that Valencia's thoughtfulness and generosity was a tender example of this all-important virtue in little souls — a virtue that Jesus looks for: the virtue of generosity.

With Stethoscope and Scapular

— 4 —

Joseph

It was now three months since we had moved out of our little white castle. The landlord had raised the rent, and Jean and I agreed that it was time to move. I had accumulated a small amount of money in our savings account, just enough for a down payment on a house, an all-brick split level rambler that we could call our own. The bottom level would serve perfectly as the future office, with enough space for two examining rooms, a bathroom and a waiting room. The entrance was a bit awkward — the patients would have to come in through a large, sliding glass door located in the rear of the house. It was a heavy door, and although adults would have no difficulty, I was concerned about the children and hoped it would present no major problem for them.

If Jean's obstetrician was correct, today was her due date, the day predicted for the birth of our baby. I was scheduled to start Saturday morning office hours in about an hour and was sitting at my desk, staring at my bookcase on the opposite wall.

Leaning back in my chair with my eyes focused on the third shelf of the bookcase, I noticed that my Mitchell and Nelson textbook on pediatrics was out of date, and I made a silent resolution to purchase the latest addition at the medical school bookstore as soon as possible.

Lost in thought, I was jolted back to the present by the sound of voices coming from the reception area. Looking at my watch, I was surprised; it was a quarter to the hour, forty-five minutes before my first patient was scheduled to arrive.

"Anybody here?" a voice yelled from the reception area.

Stepping out into the short hallway, I quickly entered the reception area. A muscular man, older than I with a butch haircut, stood ram-rod straight in the center of the room. His clean-shaven face, unfamiliar to me, was rugged and well-tanned. In his arms he held a small girl about six years of age, her face buried in his shoulder. The child was whimpering, and through a rent in her blouse I could see blood oozing from a small area between her shoulder blades. The stain seemed to be increasing in size.

"Are you the doctor?" he crisply asked.

"Yes — what happened?"

"Just five minutes ago my daughter, Julie, somehow backed into the blade of a kitchen knife that our older son had carelessly left on our sink counter."

Without even inquiring as to his name I replied, "That looks like a bad wound. Bring her right back and we'll have a look at her."

Following me into one of my two examining rooms, the man placed his daughter face down on the table. She immediately moved her head to the side and was now facing us. She was a delicate child with waxen features and silky long, black hair. Her thin lips were taut and locked in fear.

"Just try to relax, Julie," I said. "I'm going to lift up the back of your blouse to look at your cut." It was a nasty looking horizontal gash about one-and-a-half inches in length traversing the backbone area between the shoulder blades. It was still bleeding, so I grabbed some four-by-four gauze patches and applied pressure to the wound.

"Daddy, it hurts," she weakly cried.

"Don't worry, Julie," he snapped, "the doctor's going to fix you up."

"It's going to have to be sutured, Mr. ah — I'm afraid I don't even know your name."

"Bruster, Doctor, Horatio Bruster," he sharply replied.

His answers portrayed a man used to giving orders; I wondered what he did for a living.

With the baby due at any moment, Jean had not been helping me in the office. I had hired someone else, a tall gangly Scandinavian gal by the name of Olga who seemed to be working out fairly well. At the moment, however, it was just the little girl's father and me, and I saw no reason why — with a little help from him — I couldn't stitch up the wound.

"Blood doesn't bother you, does it, Mr. Bruster?"

"Master Sergeant Bruster, U.S. Marine Corps, Doctor," he replied. Then with a proud smile he added, "I'm used to blood; I was in on the Normandy landing."

"Good. I'm afraid I'm going to need your help. My office nurse isn't due in for another thirty minutes, so if you'll just hold your daughter's legs, I'll get started."

"Sure, glad to."

I drew up some xylocaine, a local anesthetic, and placed it on a small surgical tray. I placed a drape sheet over the wound, and after washing my hands, started to clean the laceration. It started to bleed more. It was a deep cut involving the tissue under the skin right down to the muscle. I glanced to my right and noticed the father was not looking at what I was doing, but was staring straight ahead, at the wall.

Julie softly cried, "Daddy, hold my hand."

"Grip the table, Julie and be brave. I have to hold your legs."

"She's being very good, Mr. Bruster. You could hold her hand if you wish."

He neither replied nor moved, so I didn't pursue my suggestion and went about my task of starting to anesthetize around the wound.

"This may hurt a bit, honey. I have to inject a little numb medicine, but it will be over in a second and then you won't feel a thing."

I jabbed the needle just under the skin and injected a bleb of anesthetic liquid. Julie squealed briefly. I noticed a movement in the father's actions and was suddenly aware that he was looking directly over my shoulder into the area of repair. When I took out the needle in order to inject it into a new location, the needle-hole started to bleed briskly. I must have hit a small capillary, because suddenly the whole lacerated area started to fill with fresh blood. I was not alarmed and knew that a little pressure was all that was needed.

What happened in the next few moments came about so quickly that I'm not sure what occurred first. I was holding a pressure dressing over the wound when suddenly I heard a loud thud. In the same moment, the father disappeared from my peripheral vision. I looked around — and finally, down — and couldn't believe my eyes. Julie's Marine daddy had fainted.

How could he do this, I thought to myself. I was just about to ask him to get some fresh gauze and relieve me by applying pressure on Julie's wound while I cracked open some suture string. But, instead, he had fainted. My first impulse was anger. Here was a Marine trained to defend us from the enemy, and he faints on me at the sight of blood. But then my anger gave way to concern and compassion; after all, it was his little daughter's blood.

"What was that noise, Daddy," whispered Julie.

"Nothing to worry about, Julie," I replied. "Just close your eyes, honey, and try to go to sleep."

"Why's Daddy lying on the floor, Doctor?"

"Julie, I'll explain later. Just close your eyes now — please!"

I grabbed some tape and quickly anchored the pressure dressing to Julie's back. Then I started attending her father. All I kept thinking was that this was a lousy way to start the day. Particularly a Saturday, and most particularly the Saturday I was scheduled to become a father.

"Sergeant, Sergeant Bruster, wake up, wake up," I shouted, slapping his cheeks. "Come on, wake up," I insisted.

His eyes started fluttering and he groaned, "What happened, what..."

"You fainted, Mr. Bruster. You told me blood didn't bother you, but you fainted. Do you feel okay?"

"Yes, yes, I'm fine," and then with a note of embarrassment he added, "Thanks."

"Just don't move. Here, let me put this pillow under your head." I grabbed a pillow from a nearby chair and thrust it under the back of his head. Just stay put for a few minutes while I take care of your daughter."

"Can I open my eyes yet?" said a little voice.

"Sure can, Julie. Your daddy is fine, but I'm going to have to fix your cut."

With the area completely anesthetized and the father now fully conscious (but resting on the floor), I was for the first time able to rivet my attention on the job at hand. For the next fifteen minutes that it took to repair the wound, Julie, pain free, was the perfect patient.

Just as I finished dressing the wound, Sergeant Horatio Bruster suddenly stood up. I noticed immediately that he was a changed man. Gone was the authoritative voice and the touch of bravado as he quietly asked, "How are you doing, little lady?"

She answered, "I'm fine, Daddy. Are you okay?"

"You're daddy is A-okay now that his little sweetheart is all fixed up." He then tenderly gathered his daughter into his arms and faced me. "Thanks, Doctor, for sewing up my little girl — and I apologize for passing out on you."

"No problem, Sergeant. I've seen it happen to more robust men than you. I'm just thankful you didn't hurt yourself."

With some instruction on home care and when to return to have the sutures removed, I said good-bye to a now-smiling Julie and a very humble Marine Master Sergeant.

I had not forgotten that Jean's due date was today, and being a compulsive and exacting physician, it never occurred to me that the baby would not be the same way and like a good fellow, enter the world on the planned day. Knowing I had to be free on this very important day, I had already made arrangements to sign out to Enrico.

Enrico Davoli, a good friend of mine since my residency days at Metropolitan Children's', had recently moved to our community and had opened his own office. In recent conversations with him it had been decided that it could be mutually advantageous if we joined forces and formed a partnership. We shared similar ideas on the practice of pediatrics, were almost the same age and worked well together.

Enrico would prove over the years to be one of the truest friends it has ever been my pleasure to know. He is a person who always could be counted on, particularly in crisis situations.

With some lab results on a patient in my right hand and a pencil in my left, I cradled the telephone between my chin and left shoulder. "Enrico, this is Joe. You haven't forgotten that I'm signing out to you, have you?"

"Forget," he chuckled, almost silently. "You must be kidding, Joe. How could I forget? Isn't Jean supposed to be having the baby today?"

"Right, today is the day. Jean has her suitcase packed, and I have the car gassed up and we are just a-waiting."

Enrico knew all about babies. His wife, Jane, had given birth to twin boys about a month earlier — and with Cecelia (their oldest child) and Frank, next in line, that made four.

"How is Jean doing, Joe?"

"Not bad; however, she keeps getting false labor pains, and they are driving me nuts. One time we were halfway to the hospital — another time actually there — before they stopped."

Enrico laughed again. "Hope you recognize the real thing when it happens, Joe."

"Yeah, I know what you mean. But anyway, back to business. Before I sign out to you, let me tell you about a sixteen-year-old boy I saw earlier this morning. Johnathan Mountgomery is his name, by the way."

While talking, I was looking at a lab sheet which contained the results of a blood count that I had obtained on Johnathan. The results were disturbing. The facts of the case as I gave them to Enrico were rather simple. The boy had had a low-grade fever for two weeks and had been getting increasingly fatigued. The physical exam revealed nothing outstanding other than a few swollen cervical and axillary lymph glands.

"It's the length of the fever, Enrico, and the blood count results that really bother me."

"Before you give me the results, Joe, let me ask you a few questions. Were the swollen glands painful?

"No, not really."

He paused, thought awhile and then asked, "What about the fever — has it been continuous or intermittent?"

"It seems to come and go, but he has at least one elevation a day."

"Hmmm, okay. Now, what about those lab results?"

"Well, this is what really concerns me. His total white cell count is very low, his platelet count is low as well — only 70,000 — and his red cells are low, too."

"Were there any abnormal white cells?"

I knew instantly what Enrico was referring to. Were there any blast forms, a hallmark of leukemia.

"None were reported, Enrico."

"What about his spleen? You said nothing, so I assume you didn't feel it."

"No, I didn't." An enlarged spleen in a leukemic could have been a bad sign, so I knew why Enrico asked.

"Joe, you know what the next step is."

"Yeah, I sure do — a bone marrow — I've already contacted a hematologist. The boy and his parents are seeing him later today and he will give you a call as soon as he has the results."

"Well, Joe, leave the rest to me and I'll take care of it. By the way, what did you tell the parents?"

"I didn't want to alarm them before we actually substantiate what is wrong, so I told them that his blood count was low and he would have to see a blood specialist who would get a special test and then possibly prescribe some medicine to get his blood count up."

"Fine. Well, you get back to your wife and don't worry about the practice. I'll take over...talk to you Monday!"

That's one of the many things I liked about my future partner. When he said he would take over and not to worry, he meant it.

I looked at my watch and noticed it was a little past noon. I had heard Jean rustling around upstairs and wondered how our mother-to-be was doing. Inserting Johnathan Mountgomery's ominous lab report into his folder, I pushed my chair back from the desk and rapidly climbed the stairs. One nice advantage about an office in the home was that it was no more than ten steps to tranquillity.

Entering the living room I noticed Jean, still in her nightgown, sitting on the sofa with her back toward me. As she turned toward me I asked, "Did you sleep well, honey?"

Putting her hand over her mouth, Jean stifled a yawn and said, "Not too bad. I had a little stomach acid that bothered me a bit, but for the most part I slept rather well and — oh! Wait a second, I did hear a loud bang very early this morning, which woke me up, but then I fell back to sleep. What was that noise, anyway?"

"That was none other than Master Sergeant Horatio Bruster keeling over in one of the exam rooms."

Jean's eyes expressed first horror, then surprise as I related all the facts.

"But you say they both left smiling?"

"Yes, I'm happy to say, they both left smiling. But no more about Sergeant Bruster; how about you? Today's the day, you know. Have you had any more of those false labor pains?"

Jean squinted her eyes as if trying to decide. "No, no, I don't think so. They always seem to hurt, but I have had some painless contractions that really confuse me."

"Well, I wouldn't pay any attention to the painless ones, honey, and I think we're experts on the false ones. They always hurt, and they never seem to last longer than a total of thirty minutes."

She didn't reply, just smiled in agreement. Jean looked so beautiful to me, sitting there on the couch. To me the most wonderful of all sights in the world is a pregnant woman, but when it's my wife — ah! That's a very special sight.

The rest of the day I puttered around the back yard cutting grass and pulling weeds. As a gardener I was young and hopeful in those early years and ever in search of the last dandelion. My dad prided himself on his emerald green carpet that surrounded our home when I was a child. I guess my subconscious was always trying to catch up to him. Every now and then I went inside the house to see how Jean was doing and if anything was happening. She was spending a quiet day reading, resting and waiting. But nothing, absolutely nothing had happened, was happening or would happen that day.

It was already about 11:00 that night and we were both getting ready for bed when I asked, "Gee, honey, are you sure you and your obstetrician counted right?"

George McDonald, her doctor, was my obstetrical gynecology resident when I was an intern at Granger General. He was an ideal physician: friendly, able and always optimistic. We had great confidence in him.

"What did George say the last time you saw him?"

My question took her by surprise, since I had asked it only about twenty times in the past month.

"You know as well as I what he said. Today is the day."

Looking at her I shook my head. I knew one thing for sure. The lad was not adhering to the master plan. Playfully and ever so gently I rapped on Jean's tummy and said, "Son, this is your daddy speaking; you do understand that today is the day, don't you..."

He obviously didn't, and already was exerting his independence. The next three days were even quieter than Jean's due date. There was not even a twitch or a ripple from his uterine home. Oh, sure, he was squirming around enough, but he wasn't going to leave.

By Tuesday we almost forgot he was there. My future partner was on stand-by to take over the practice the moment Jean went into labor. I had talked to Enrico earlier that day and he had given me the latest news on Johnathan Mountgomery. His low blood count was not the result of leukemia, but was caused by an overwhelming viral infection. This was great news because the prognosis for full recovery was excellent. I audibly breathed a sigh of relief and reminded Enrico that Jean and I wanted him to be the baby's pediatrician.

The remainder of the day passed uneventfully with few problem patients, and before we knew it, it was time to retire. Climbing into bed, we needed only a sheet to cover us. It was hot and sticky outside, and even the chirping crickets and belching frogs sounded sluggish. In fact, all the voices of the night were performing in slow motion — with the exception of a happy mockingbird who had taken refuge in the branches of a birch tree directly outside one of the bedroom windows. For the past two weeks he had been gaily serenading us practically every night.

Turning out the lights, I put my arm around Jean and asked, "Anything happening, honey?"

She snuggled close and whispered, "Nothing, absolutely nothing. But I know he's getting stronger."

I whispered back, "Oh, why do you say that?"

"His kick; it's ferocio*us,*" she said out loud.

"I think he finally wants out, honey. Might be a good sign."

Just then our caroler started a melodious repertoire. He first started with a cat bird cry, followed by a robin red breast ditty and then climaxed his outburst with a thrush and warbler ensemble.

"He's really full of himself tonight, isn't he," Jean remarked.

"I'll say, and louder than usual." Just then I had an idea. If mocking birds can imitate other birds, I wonder if they can imitate humans.

"Watch this, honey." I started whistling, "Rock A Bye Baby" and kept whistling it about three minutes or so. Our little friend was obviously interested, because he stopped his song. Then I stopped. After a minute or two of silence, much to our delight, he started singing in perfect pitch the melody to "Rock A Bye Baby." He kept this up for maybe three or four minutes, and then — the concert over — flew away. Soon after, we both fell asleep.

It must have been about 4:00 AM or thereabouts when I was suddenly awakened by a loud, screeching metallic noise. I bolted upright in bed and was momentarily disorientated. Jean also had been awakened and asked me what the noise was; I replied that it sounded like tires skidding just outside our front door. After a few seconds of unearthly silence another noise, louder than the first, erupted. It sounded like the roaring clatter of a powerful engine. My eardrums were ringing and my heart was pounding.

I squeezed Jean's hand. "It's coming from the front of the house. I'll investigate."

"Be careful, honey."

As I started for the front door I heard a third noise, but this time it was distant and fading. I opened the front door, stepped outside and stood on our bottom front step, which gave me a clear view of the entire street. It was empty, dark and very quiet. I wondered for a moment if it all had been a bad dream.

Returning to bed, I chatted with Jean about the strange occurrence — which she told me had frightened our child, judging by the way he was kicking up a storm.

About five minutes passed and we were just settling down when suddenly another roar, more deafening than the others, tore through the humid silence. This time it was coming from the rear of the house. We sat upright and instinctively turned in the direction of the noise. Kneeling on our pillows with our hands clutching the headboard, we looked out our rear bedroom window. An expanse of fenceless back lawns separated our house from the unoccupied houses that lined the perimeter of a cul-de-sac directly behind us. What I saw I couldn't believe. I kept rubbing my eyes, trying to wash the image away. There at a distance of 100 yards or so and headed right toward us was a large motorized vehicle, bouncing and bobbing along on an undulating desert of invisible grass.

It absolutely made no sense. The thought passed through my mind that I was in the middle of a nightmare and that a tank commander was on the march in an invincible giant tank, which was rapidly advancing on a trajectory that would propel him right through our reception area's sliding glass door.

The gleam of the high-beam headlights, which were moving through a 30-degree vertical arc, reflected off Jean's face. Mouth open, eyes disbelieving, she shouted, "What is happening? Who is in that thing?"

"I don't have the slightest idea, but if he doesn't change directions he's going to push our whole waiting room right through the front of the house into the street."

He was less than fifteen yards from our rear door, and our muscles tensed as we waited for the sound of splintering glass. "R-r-r-r-r-, r-r-r-r-..." No sound of splintering glass. At the last moment, in a sudden outflanking maneuver, the mystery driver had turned and swished through a narrow alley of grass between our house and our next-door neighbors'.

Jean and I, both too shocked to say anything, headed for the front door. Jean stood in the doorway trembling as I, in my pajamas, ran outside. The street was well-lighted and there was a full moon. Our front lawn looked like a battlefield. Huge parallel tread marks were deeply etched into the whole length of the lawn. Across the street, our neighbor's two small dogwood trees, uprooted and lying flat on the ground, had fallen victim to the mad marauder.

Jean by now was by my side and we surveyed the damage. "Just look what that maniac did to our lawn."

"Honey, you shouldn't be out here. Forget the lawn for now and let's get inside. I'll call the police."

Approximately fifteen minutes later a patrol car, red light flashing, drove into our driveway. Jean insisted on coming outside with me to talk with him. I explained to the officer the bizarre events of the past thirty minutes. He knew immediately what we were talking about and gave us the answer to our 4:00 AM riddle. Some of the local high school boys were doing what they termed "lawn jobs." They first stripped down a beat-up second hand car by removing the muffler and the original tires, then substituted wide-treaded oversized tires. In the wee hours of the morning they indiscriminately drove their vehicles over any lawn they felt like. It was vandalism, pure and simple. The officer reassured us that it was not the pattern of the hoodlums to return to the same area; however, the success rate of catching the culprits was poor. He took a vandalism report and left.

Jean and I returned to the house and sat on the living room sofa trying to decide whether it was worthwhile to go back to bed. While talking it over, I noticed that Jean suddenly winced as if in pain.

"What's wrong?" I asked.

"I'm not sure, but I think it's those false labor pains. They 've started up again."

"How long have you been having them?"

"They started about fifteen minutes ago, but this is the first really painful one."

She got up off the couch and started slowly pacing back and forth across the bare living room floor. (We had not yet purchased a carpet.)

"Are they getting stronger, honey?"

She didn't answer, but with a grim look shook her head "Yes."

I put my arm around her shoulder and we both started pacing. I kept thinking that they were false labor pains and would stop in a moment.

"Oh," she said, "these really hurt and seem to be lasting longer...I wonder..."

"I think I'd better call George."

From the description of the contractions, George told us it sounded like Jean was in early labor and we should leave immediately for the hospital. That was all we needed to hear. We flew into action. Jean grabbed, between pains, a few last-minute things from the bedroom while I snatched the over-night bag. In a few minutes we were out of the driveway and on our way.

It was about 5:30 AM and the trip without morning traffic was accomplished in less than half the normal travel time. If there had been any lingering doubts on my part, they were erased by the time we reached the hospital. Jean's pains were growing more intense and lasting longer. She squeezed my hand with each contraction and groaned. I guided her up the few steps into the emergency room, where George was waiting with a wheelchair. His easy yet concerned smile was a welcome relief to Jean as we both helped her into the chair.

"I don't have to examine her, Joe. Jean is in labor. Why don't you go sit in the third floor father's waiting room while I wheel her up to labor and delivery." Then after allowing me time for a quick kiss and an affectionate squeeze, he whisked her off to the delivery suite.

The next few hours were tense. The usual thoughts of an expectant father, in addition to those of a physician, paraded through my mind. Would the delivery be uncomplicated? How was Jean doing, how was she handling the pain? I remembered a viral infection she had when she was about three or four months pregnant. I wondered if it had had any effect on the baby. Would he have all his fingers and toes?

The seconds became minutes, the minutes hours as I tried to get my mind on more pleasant thoughts. I read the newspaper for the third time and still couldn't tell anyone what the headlines were. It must have been about 9:30 or 10:00 AM and I was fumbling with the sports page when a smiling George entered the fathers' waiting room and extended his hand toward me and said, "Congratulations, Joe. You're the father of a healthy eight-pound baby boy." It is difficult to describe the emotion that welled up inside me at that moment, but it was one of the most wonderful moments of my life. I was ecstatic.

It was only a short time later that I was looking at my son for the first time. I kept thinking, "Wow! This is amazing, Jean and I really did this." And he was a handsome lad, no doubt about that.

During the next few days Jean and I carried on as though we were the only parents who had ever had a son. She glowed with happiness, repeating over and over, "Isn't he beautiful! Just look at those eyes! They are so blue! And that hair, would you call it red or just rusty?"

Enrico checked him over and assured us he was a very healthy boy. His stay in the hospital was uneventful; he ate ravenously and slept soundly. On the third day we headed for home. Jean had dressed him in an all-blue outfit, and on his head he had a small peaked hat. On the way home from the hospital I had a difficult time paying attention to my driving. I kept looking at Jean and little Joseph. Jean kept cooing and talking like all new mothers, and I kept up a low-grade chuckle the entire trip home.

I guess Joe was destined to be a physician. As a toddler he liked parading around the house with my stethoscope draped around his neck, and when he was older he enjoyed making house calls and going to the hospital with me. Even when very, very young he had the gift of sympathy. Two of his best friends were my partner's twin sons. I recall one Sunday afternoon Jean and I, together with Joseph, were visiting Enrico, Jane and their children. On this particular occasion one of the twins took a nasty fall and Joe instinctively toddled over to him, put his arm around him and comforted him.

The summer before he applied to medical school, Joe worked as an orderly at County General and thoroughly enjoyed it. On his admission letter to the various medical schools to which he applied there was a question asking why he wanted to enter the medical profession. Joe said, "This past summer I secured a job as a transportation aide at County General which presented an opportunity for direct daily patient contact. I know what it is to be sick, having had infectious mononucleosis for a large part of my last semester in college. This illness and my work at the hospital have made me realize just how lucky I am to be healthy. My heart goes out to those who aren't as fortunate. Each morning before going to work, I made a commitment to try to cheer up the patients that I saw during the day. I especially remember one morning when I was wheeling a cancer patient back to his room. This man appeared to be out of touch with reality due to his medication and illness. However, I still felt I had to do something for him, and so I carried on a monologue with him all the way to his room. After getting him into bed I said good-bye and expected no response, but to my surprise and joy, he said in a strained voice, "Thank you." This man died a week later. I never will see this man again, but he did something for me for which I wish I could have thanked him. He made me see that this was the profession in which I belong.

Joe was accepted at Georgetown Medical School, passed his boards in Internal Medicine, and just this summer he completed his fellowship in Oncology Hematology. At present he, his wife Barbara and their two children, Taylor and Ryan, are living in Richmond, where he has recently joined a group practice in Oncology. His mother and I think he is a very competent and caring doctor who is going to help a great many people. Jean and I thank God for our son Joe.

— 5 —

The Prayer

Saint Therese of the Child Jesus was a late nineteenth-century Carmelite nun who died of tuberculosis when only twenty-four years old. She was the saint of the "little way," which was described by her biographers as a path paved by continuous acts of love toward God and neighbor. She used to say, "If I pick up a pin from the floor and do it out of love for God, it has great merit." For to Therese, the smallest act of pure love was of more value than mighty acts done without this noble intention. Unsaid but surely implied was the fact that someone else would be spared from having to pick up the pin.

I was standing like any father outside the nursery window, proudly staring at our newly born daughter, Mary Ann. I recalled Saint Therese's "little way" and the thought occurred to me that I would have liked to have canonized the sweet young nurse who tenderly moved Mary Ann's tiny hand that had been awkwardly flexed against the incubator wall. I knew it was hurting Mary Ann, and the nurse — God bless her — realized it also.

Mary Ann was born seven weeks premature and only weighed four and a half pounds. She seemed lively the first few hours after birth; however now, at five hours old, her respirations had increased. I was disturbed over this development, but not overly alarmed. After all, it was not uncommon for premature infants to have some breathing problems which, in my experience, resolved themselves quickly.

Jean was standing beside me, and I had placed my arm around her waist. Without looking at me she said, "Isn't she beautiful, darling?"

Turning toward her I squeezed her hand and replied, "Just like her mother."

Jean, pale and tired, managed a half smile and then quizzically asked, "She's breathing so fast, are you sure she is going to be okay?"

"Honey," I replied, "I've treated maybe a half dozen babies with this problem before and they all, after a few rocky days, have done well."

"What does Enrico think?"

"He feels the same way. He is going to start an intravenous infusion to give her fluids, calories and electrolytes. Her color is basically good, but because she is a little blue around the mouth he is giving her oxygen."

Sadly Jean thought aloud, "If only I could go inside and hold her in my arms, just for a moment."

We both knew that was impossible. Mary Ann needed the help the incubator was giving her. She had the signs and symptoms of early Hyaline Membrane disease, a mysterious illness that had a predilection for premature babies. The disease was caused by the lack of a vital chemical needed for proper lung expansion of the terminal air sacs. This chemical, under normal circumstances, took form in developing babies' lungs late in pregnancy. Following birth, without the chemical the terminal air sacs started collapsing and an insidious membrane developed inside the lungs called a hyaline membrane. This membrane, coupled with the collapsing air sacs, prevents life-giving oxygen from reaching the blood stream.

The membrane was forming inside our little baby's lungs.

I walked Jean slowly back to her room, once again reassuring her that Mary Ann would recover. As soon as I finished with the patients scheduled for that afternoon I would return, I promised Jean.

Back in the office I found it difficult to concentrate. Fortunately, the nurse-receptionist had canceled all the well check-ups and I only had to attend to sick patients and rechecks. I was tense the whole afternoon and couldn't wait to return to the hospital to be with Mary Ann and Jean.

I was relieved when the last patient departed. Hastily I scribbled a note on the chart, said good-bye to the nurse-receptionist, switched off the light and left.

As I backed out the driveway the feeling of tension mounted. I had not even inquired about Joseph, who was being cared for by our next-door neighbor. I knew Jean would ask, and I mentally admonished myself for having forgotten. Driving over to the hospital I kept thinking to myself that Mary Ann had to be improving, she just had to be.

With home-bound traffic going in the opposite direction, I was at the Medical Center Hospital in record time. After parking the car I quickly navigated the hospital's front steps — and not even waiting for the elevator, I raced up the three flights of stairs to the nursery. Entering the nursing alcove, I immediately recognized through the nursery window my future partner, Enrico, listening with his stethoscope to Mary Ann's lungs through one of the incubator portholes.

I quickly gowned, masked and washed my hands. With the stethoscope ear prongs in his ears, Enrico did not hear me as I approached the incubator. It had been five hours since I last saw Mary Ann. Looking over Enrico's left shoulder, my heart sank. She was decidedly worse. Her skin was a mottled blue, her body limp and her chest was heaving up and down more rapidly than ever.

I tapped Enrico on the shoulder and we exchanged a few words on the struggling baby's condition. "She's really struggling, Joe, but she is a fighter," Enrico noted. I appreciated his optimism. For a few moments we discussed changes in oxygen flow and fluid orders that he was making in an attempt to help her. I felt crushed by Mary Ann's turn for the worse, but Enrico's presence, concern and the changes he was making in treatment were encouraging.

I had yet to talk to Jean about the gravity of Mary Ann's condition, and I dreaded it. I left Enrico with our baby and slowly went down the outside corridor toward my wife's room. Entering the room, I caught a glimpse of her beautiful smile before she saw me. She must have been thinking about our new little daughter and the dresses she was going to clothe her in. My first impulse was to leave, but the moment had to be faced.

As she looked in my direction her smile disappeared. My looks betrayed my thoughts. I walked over to her bed and sat down on it, taking her hands in mine. "Darling, I..."

Before I could finish, Jean replied, "Mary Ann's not doing well, is she?"

"No, no, she isn't; her breathing is very rapid and her color is not good."

"What does Enrico think?"

"He's concerned, but he said she is a real fighter and that is in her favor."

With the knowledge of Mary Ann's strong desire to live, over the next few minutes we consoled and fortified each other and resolved not to yield to despair. It was so important to have hope, even in the face of impending tragedy. The hour was late and I told Jean that she must sleep. She pleaded with me, "You'll let me know the moment anything happens, regardless what it is, won't you, darling?"

"I will, honey, I promise I'll be right by your side the moment there is any change."

Kissing her tears away, I left.

It was three AM when Enrico called to tell me that Mary Ann had died. I remember the moment as though it were yesterday. I had fallen asleep on the living room couch fully clothed with the belief that if she lived until morning she would survive. When the phone rang I knew who it was and what he would tell me. I was numbed by the news. I did not immediately cry; I couldn't — it was so strange. I didn't understand my feelings at the time. I remembered my promise to Jean. The return to the hospital, the slow walk to the third floor, the entrance into her room, all were so painful.

Jean was sobbing deeply as I held her close to me. "Oh, no, no, no, it can't be, it can't be," she kept repeating over and over.

"Sweetheart, sweetheart," I replied, "she fought, she fought so hard, but her little lungs just couldn't do it."

Jean's sobs were heartbreaking. I squeezed her closer to me, smothering her sobs.

"Enrico and the nursing staff did everything they could. Enrico was with her all the while, darling."

"I know, I know."

"He had the priest baptize her earlier this evening."

"Good, good, I'm glad he did that. Enrico is such a good friend."

Mary Ann's funeral service was a simple one, and only the few friends who knew of our tragedy came. The casket, all white and only two feet long, was with great respect placed by the two pallbearers at the foot of the altar. The priest said some beautiful and consoling words on the Beatific Vision that our innocent baptized daughter now enjoyed; but the church, so cold and empty, seemed to reflect the coldness and emptiness of our own hearts. It was the warmth of our friends who had come to the service and were to visit us afterwards that acted as a healing balm to our wounded spirits. Our next door neighbor's elderly mother came to the service just to let us know she cared. Her painful, arthritic steps slowly mounting the church steps live to this day in my memory.

Only two cars made up the funeral procession, which ended in a far corner of the cemetery. Mary Ann was buried in a small grave near a dogwood tree. Her marker was a simple bronze plaque, six by eighteen inches. It had a picture of Jesus etched on it welcoming little children into His open arms. It was difficult returning home to the empty bassinet and the clothes we had bought in anticipation of bringing Mary Ann home.

Heart-wrenching days followed. We both were young and full of promise and never had experienced a death of a loved one that was so close and meaningful to us. It was doubly difficult for Jean, who had carried Mary Ann in her womb for over seven months. A much stronger bond than my own had developed; Jean had felt Mary Ann's movements and had, mentally, tenderly held her many times in her arms.

It was once again the compassion and concern of friends and acquaintances that continued the healing process. Dr. Arthur, my friendly competitor in our community, dropped over late one evening shortly after Mary Ann's burial. He said he was on his way back from the hospital and just wanted to express his condolences. I'm sure he was tired and anxious to go home, yet he visited with us for about an hour or so. Another sweet person, a woman whose four children were patients of mine, with a heart as big as her smile brought over a freshly baked apple pie not a day after hearing about Mary Ann's death. Enrico and his good wife, Jane, were by our side whenever possible.

As one week followed another our depression lessened, and finally, when Jean became pregnant again, our spirits soared. Within less than a year after Mary Ann's death, on a morning late in April, Cathy was born. She also arrived early, but she was not as premature as Mary Ann and was a pound and a half heavier. Cathy had a strong cry and I was confident that all would be well. Yet not all was well, for within twenty-four hours after her birth the same mysterious membrane, with its suffocating power, had started to form inside Cathy's lungs.

As a physician I was frustrated and had never encountered or even heard of a family having had successive children with Hyaline Membrane disease. As a father I was devastated. Its relentless grip could not be pried loose, and slowly but surely the life ebbed from our beautiful little daughter.

We buried little Cathy next to her tiny sister Mary Ann. A similar bronze plaque with an identical etching of the welcoming Lord was placed over her grave. A second dogwood tree would soon be planted. What words could describe our anguish. What words of comfort could I possibly offer to my poor Jean.

Once again our friends came to our rescue. What seemed impossible at first they made possible as family and friends soothed our freshly opened wound.

I recall the day after Cathy's death, sitting in the car. It seemed as though the world were coming apart around me and I cried, half screamed aloud, like a five-year-old child: "God, God, why are You doing this to us, what terrible sin have I committed that You wish to torture and punish us so." My faith had long ago taught me to believe that God had a purpose behind everything, but that morning I could not even begin to understand what it could possibly be.

Barely a year after Cathy's death, Jean became pregnant again. It was for the fourth time in a little less than four years. It was a surprise pregnancy, and we were unprepared as to what to do. For some reason which I could not explain, neither of us were discouraged. In fact, we both were determined that everything possible that could be done, had to be done to protect this pregnancy. I haunted medical libraries searching the medical literature for every scrap of information on Hyaline Membrane disease I could find. My efforts were rewarded when I found one particular article that sounded very encouraging. In Buffalo, New York, my home town, at Children's Hospital a group of doctors were doing studies on babies with Hyaline Membrane disease using an enzyme called streptokinase. The enzyme was believed to possess the capability to dissolve the membrane and save babies who had the disease. The whole study was still experimental, but the results were most promising. I called the doctor in charge of the study and told him of our problem. I remember the conversation well and recall asking him, "Doctor, if my wife and I decide to temporarily move to Buffalo during the final weeks of her pregnancy and if she goes once again into labor prematurely, will you include our baby in your study?"

"Dr. Evers, we sure hope your wife carries the baby to term, but if she does not and she delivers at our hospital we would be pleased to include the baby in the study."

With this reassuring news it was settled that we would move to Buffalo in mid-November and stay with my parents until Jean delivered.

It was in September of this same year that Enrico and I officially formed our partnership, and I felt badly having to ask him to cover the combined practice for eight or more weeks. His answer didn't surprise me at all: "Joe, don't worry about it, it's the only thing you and Jean can possibly think of doing. I'll take care of the practice."

"But old buddy, I worry about how you can handle a double practice for eight weeks alone."

"Don't worry about it, Joe; if I get tired I'll get coverage from some of our pediatrician friends. We have lots of them, you know."

That was just like Enrico. I have often thought to myself that Enrico Davoli should be a synonym in Webster's dictionary for the phrase "true friend." He is that special person who is always there when a serious need arises. He always answers the call.

In mid-November the three of us — Jean, two-and-a-half-year-old Joseph and myself — moved northward to Buffalo. My parents, both wonderful people, welcomed us with open arms and made their home ours. When we arrived, the city — true to its reputation as the refrigerator of the north — already had six inches of snow on the ground. Joseph was delighted, and he squealed with joy as the three of us had gentle snowball wars with each other. The Buffalo workout must have helped, for in latter years he would pitch for his little league baseball team and quarterback for his boys' club football team.

After each snowfall we enjoyed taking long wintry walks up one street and down the other outside my parents' home. One particular morning after an unusually heavy snowfall, the snow was

piled so high along each side of the street that the three-foot reflectors used to mark the end of each driveway were all but covered up.
We were briskly walking along, I a little ahead of Jean, who was
holding one of Joe's hands. We noticed as we walked that Joe was
fascinated by the red reflectors and kept pointing at them and saying, "Lookum Pop, lookum Pop." He never called me Pop, so I was
a little confused as to what he was trying to tell us. I fell back
alongside Jean, a masterful interpreter of toddler and little child
language, and asked, "Honey, what is he trying to tell us?"

Before she could answer Joe broke Jean's grip and quickly
crawled on all fours up a snow bank with his eye fixed on the top of
the mound of snow where six inches of the pole with its red reflector jutted out. Reaching the summit of what must have looked to
him like a miniature mountain, Joe grabbed the pole with both hands
and with his face right up to the reflector started licking it.

"I knew that's what he was thinking," laughed Jean. "He thinks
it's a red lollipop. Oh, look at his face...the cold reflector must
have nipped his tongue."

I wish I could have captured on film the expression of surprise
and disgust that registered on Joe's face. I knew that the cold stung
his tongue, but the situation was so funny. Little children are so
innocent and so honest in their responses and actions. Being a parent has so many great moments.

The days slipped by one after the other and we adjusted rapidly to our new surroundings. I visited all my old school friends
and introduced Jean and Joe to them. It was refreshing to renew
old friendships. More importantly, as the days passed by the baby
inside Jean's womb matured a tiny bit more each day.

Every evening at a certain hour, while Jean was resting upstairs, I retreated to my parents' basement recreation room. It was
a tiled room with a rug, several chairs and a couch. It was a warm
room, a room filled with memories. It was here on many occasions while in high school and college that my buddies and I would
gather for pinochle or poker games. Stories would be swapped
and laughs shared.

It was also a quiet room, ideal for prayer and reflection. It was
here that I chose to kneel on the tiled floor for thirty minutes each
evening and pray to God, the Author of all life. My prayer was a
simple one; it was a dialogue with God. I would say over and over

again, sometimes aloud, sometimes in a whisper, sometimes in thought only: "Dear God, you know how much Jean and I love You; we want only to do Your will. You and You alone are the Author of all life; You gave us Mary Ann for a few hours and then You took her to Yourself; You took her home. You then gave us Cathy for a short while and then gathered her into Your loving arms. Now Jean is pregnant again and we want this child very, very much. What is Your will for us?"

I then would imagine Our Heavenly Father, God, holding out both His arms. In one arm He was handing a little baby to Jean and myself. In the other He was drawing a little baby unto Himself. In my imagination He then would say to me, "Joe, you can choose whatever arm you want. What do you wish?"

My answer was always the same, "No, dear Father, You know best. You decide; Jean and I will accept whatever You choose for us."

I had devised a calendar in which I kept track of the very hours of Jean's pregnancy. Knowing the probable day she had conceived, it was not difficult to calculate that mid-January was the target date for the delivery of a healthy term baby.

By early December we both were feeling quite confident and had decided to go out to dinner at a nearby restaurant and celebrate. We had something to celebrate: Jean looked great, her spirits were high, and more important — her most recent visit to the obstetrician revealed that the baby was thriving within her quiet uterus. It was a pleasant family-style restaurant, and our table was near a cozy fireplace with a blazing fire. A Christmas wreath with a beautiful red bow hung over the fireplace beneath a spacious mantle. On top of the mantle, flanking one side of the wreath, were three tall red candles. On the other side was a manger with the adoring shepherds and animals surrounding the Holy Family. Looking at the manger, thoughts of the coming Christ-child and our own baby flooded my mind. I think Jean must have been thinking similar thoughts.

"How many days is it now, Darling?" Jean asked inquisitively.

"Well, it's ten days until Christmas and..." looking at my watch I replied, "it's two hundred and four days, nine hours and thirty-three minutes that you've been pregnant."

She laughed her sweet laugh and said, "You're kidding me — you can't have it figured out that exactly!"

I winked at her and replied, "Well, maybe I'm off by a few hours, but not by much more. One thing I know for sure, we need about another month to feel completely safe."

It had been a happy evening, thinking and talking about the coming Christmas and about our own blessed event. We had just about finished desert when suddenly I noticed a pained expression on Jean's face.

"What's wrong?"

"I'm not sure, but I think I just had a labor pain." We just stared at each other for the next few seconds, too stunned to say anything.

"Maybe it's just one of those false labor pains you used to get when you were pregnant with Joseph."

She winced again and replied, "We'd better leave; I just had another one."

We left quickly and said nothing to each other going home in the car. Periodically glancing at Jean's face, I could tell each time she had a pain. Once getting home, I immediately placed a call to the obstetrician who was caring for her. I told him how often each pain was occurring and how long it was lasting. He listened carefully and then replied that it could be early labor and advised us to leave at once for the hospital, where an obstetrical resident would examine Jean. Without a moment's hesitation I helped her pack an overnight bag and we left for the hospital.

It was a cold, silent night, disturbed only by a gentle snowfall. The streets were plowed, and there were few cars traveling as we headed down Main Street toward Children's Hospital. I kept looking at Jean, hoping the pains would stop. She knew exactly what I was thinking and kept shaking her head from side to side, indicating that they had not.

"How often are they coming?" I asked.

"About every few minutes."

Judging from her pained expression, they seemed to be lasting about twenty to thirty seconds. I gunned the accelerator about the same time that a patrol car with two policemen inside pulled up along side of us. I opened my window, and the policeman on the passenger side yelled at me, "What do you think you're doing; don't you realize you're over the speed limit?"

I yelled back, "My wife's having a baby! Can you give me an escort to Children's Hospital?"

"Glad to — follow us!" and with the light flashing they pulled in front of our car and led the way.

A scant ten minutes later an attendant was wheeling Jean into the maternity ward. I followed behind the wheelchair in close pursuit. A nurse intercepted me as I attempted to enter the examination room with my wife.

Surprised by my boldness she said, "I'm sorry, Sir, you can't go in there."

"But I'm a doctor and that's my wife, and I would like to be with her."

"I'm sorry, Doctor, but it's hospital policy that the husband — even if a physician — cannot be present while the obstetrical resident is interviewing your wife."

"I understand," I replied, "but could I speak to the doctor as soon as he completes his exam?"

"Certainly."

Reluctantly I sat in a chair just outside the examination room, anxiously awaiting what would happen next. The obstetrical resident had already entered the room, so I knew it would be just a matter of time before the door opened and we would know whether Jean was in labor. When you're waiting for monumental news it seems as though it takes forever. My feelings at the moment are hard to describe; I knew that if Jean were in labor, the baby would not be able to escape hyaline membrane formation. Jean would be delivering at about the same time she had given birth to the other two babies. We then would be at the mercy of the experimental drug. However, I also kept hoping that maybe, just maybe she was not in labor and they were just unusually strong false labor pains.

I kept staring at that door and clutching the rosary beads in my pocket. Finally the door opened and the young doctor emerged. He immediately headed in my direction.

"Dr. Evers, my name is Leo Anderson. I'm the second year obstetrical resident and I've just completed my examination of your wife, and..."

I interrupted him before he could finish. "Is she in labor, Doctor? That's all I want to know, is she in labor?"

"Well, your wife's cervix is one to two centimeters dilated, Doctor. Her pains are fairly regular and painful and, and...yes, I believe she is in early labor."

I said nothing, but with head down and resigned to whatever awaited us sighed a long sigh.

"I'm sorry, Dr. Evers; I wish I could tell you something different. Mrs. Evers told me about the terrible tragedies you both have had with her last two pregnancies."

Nodding in agreement I replied, "May I see her, Dr. Anderson?"

"If you could just wait a few minutes the nurse will be taking her to a room in the delivery suite."

I said nothing in reply, but left the waiting area I had been in and stepped outside into a corridor. I slowly paced up and down the corridor and for the next fifteen minutes and prayed the Rosary. I then entered the maternity suite, went to the nurse's station and asked the nurse what room my wife was in. She gave me the number, and with measured steps I entered her room. Jean was in her night garments, lying under a blanket. We just looked at each other. No words were necessary.

"Are they getting worse?"

"I'm having one right now; here, give me your hand." With that she took my hand and placed it on her abdomen. I felt through my fingertips her rigid uterine contraction and was convinced she was in early labor.

The nurse entered the room and asked that I leave. I didn't want to, but reluctantly obeyed. Alone outside the maternity suite I suddenly felt terrified at the possible consequences and could only think of finding some quiet place to pray. It was an automatic response. Prayer is something I have done since a child. It is a habit fostered in me by my parents.

I found a small empty waiting room off the maternity suite which was dark and quiet. I recall falling to my knees, and using my own words, praying as I had never prayed before in my life. My prayer was from the deepest recesses of my heart. "Dear Father, I beg Thee, please through the intercession of Thy dear Son, Jesus, and out of love for the Immaculate Heart of His Mother Mary, please — I beg Thee — give us this baby." I kept repeating this prayer over and over, using different words but with the same meaning.

After some ten to fifteen minutes I felt compelled to return to Jean's room, and only hoped I could escape the nurse's eye. The nurse was attending another patient as I entered the room. The room was dark except for a night light which faintly illuminated Jean's face. Approaching the bedside, I stood beside her, staring at her face. She was not aware of my presence and seemed to be asleep. I said nothing, but just stood there — my heart pounding — looking at her. Jean continued to sleep peacefully. After about seven minutes or so I whispered the question I almost dared not to ask: "Honey, how are you doing?"

With that she aroused and groggily replied, "Oh, is that you, honey; I must have fallen asleep. The pains, they — they seem to have stopped."

I felt an indescribable rush of joy flooding my whole body and answered, "Are you sure?"

"Yes, I haven't had one since you left the room."

Jean fell asleep as she answered. I knew the nurse must have given her a sedative, and she was exhausted from her three hours of labor. She didn't hear me, but I silently wept — in thanksgiving and joy.

The next morning Jean was discharged from the hospital, and until Sharon's delivery in the second week of January she did not have another painful contraction.

It is difficult even now to describe the joy we experienced the morning Sharon was born. The flow of happiness on Jean's face as she held Sharon in her arms is something that I had waited over two years to see. We both had waited so long, but looking at our healthy, seven-pound full-term daughter, we knew in our hearts that all would be well.

Three days later we brought Sharon home. She experienced no problems at all while in the hospital and actually had gained an ounce by the time she was discharged.

Sharon was a soft, gentle baby with very dark eyes and long, tapering fingers that rested lightly on her mother's shoulder. Looking at Sharon's fingers, I envisioned a future concert pianist.

No two parents could be happier with the indescribable gift of life that God had given to us. Over the years we would witness Sharon develop into a mature, attractive, caring young woman.

Following in her mother's footsteps, she pursued a nursing career and just recently graduated from our State University. She worked briefly this past summer for my partner and me as our office nurse. I may be a tad prejudiced in my assessment, but in all honesty I think she is one of the most conscientious nurses I have had the pleasure to work with. Frequently over the years I would hold her close and let her know she was "my most favorite daughter."

God is never outdone in generosity, and over the next three years following Sharon's birth He gave us two more healthy, beautiful daughters.

Lisa, petite and sparkly-eyed, was born fourteen months after Sharon. From the day of her birth Lisa was a dynamo of activity. Whereas baby Sharon would gently touch her mother's hair while being held, little Lisa would firmly grab it and give it a hardy yank. She had boundless energy, and it needed an outlet. Unharnessed at first, over the years it has been nicely channeled into that unique virtue called industry. Lisa always gives her best effort to every task she encounters and never starts something that she does not finish.

Lisa will graduate this summer with a degree in teacher's education and plans a career in primary education. She loves children and will make an excellent teacher. This past summer Lisa did some practice teaching in our community, and several of my small patients were her students. I was one proud father as each of the parents told me how much their child enjoyed Lisa as their teacher. Frequently over the years I have let Lisa know she is "my most favorite daughter."

Tara, our joy girl and our youngest, was born about two years after Lisa. She had her mother's large, expressive eyes, but her bubbly smile and explosive laughter were uniquely Tara's. Blessed with an easy-going temperament, she has always been a very happy person — the type of person that friends and acquaintances would say of, "Gee, Tara's such fun to be around." Her ability to find humor in just about any circumstance and project his humor gives anybody a boost just being in her company.

Even when facing adversity, she can find humor in the event. On one occasion she was the sole driver in a serious car accident which resulted in her tongue being seriously lacerated. So bad was the injury that forty stitches were required to repair it. While being transported to the hospital by ambulance, she was unable to communicate with the ambulance attendant; but knowing sign language, she tried using it. Tara tells the story best: "Can you imagine, Mom and Dad; there I was, lying on the stretcher with my mouth full of blood, and the ambulance attendant starts asking me questions like, 'Where are you hurt most, young lady?' and 'What is your name?'"

Tara laughingly continues, "Of course I didn't want all this blood rolling down my face, so I started using sign language. Then do you know what he did," Tara laughs uproariously as she continues her story, "he takes a small microphone in his hand, switches it on and says to the ambulance driver in the front, 'Say, we have a deaf girl back here, do either of you up front know sign language?" We all laugh at this point in her story.

Many times I put my arm around Tara and loudly whisper so her other two sisters can hear, "You know, Tara, you're my most favorite daughter."

Mary Ann and Cathy's death, as tragic as they are, nonetheless increased in me a spiritual awareness of God's design in our lives and the reason behind some of what at first seem to be unexplainable events.

Surely one of the greatest tragedies that can occur to parents is the unexpected death of one of their children due to an incurable disease or accident. Because of my own daughters' deaths I have discovered throughout the years I have been in practice that I have been able to emotionally identify with the parents and the bereavement ordeal they must pass through. Also, I am able to comfort them and offer them hope in a way that I do not believe, but for Mary Ann and Cathy's brief existence, I would be able to otherwise provide.

Their deaths also taught me the wisdom behind the old adage, "Work as though everything depended upon yourself; pray as though everything depends upon God." Another lesson I learned was an increased awareness in God's daily blessings and our need to offer Him praise and thanksgiving for these daily occurrences.

I recall the morning of Sharon's birth, that one of the first things I did after checking on her condition in the nursery was to find a nearby Catholic church. I was fortunate in finding one a few blocks from Children's Hospital, and I was just in time for the first morning Mass. Never was a father more thankful to his Creator than I was that morning. I poured out my heart to our sweet Saviour in my morning Communion, thanking Him over and over for our dear daughter. I have tried to keep this moment alive and particularly the special feeling of thanksgiving I experienced that morning. I do this because it is so often that I take God's blessings for granted, forgetting the Giver and the love behind His daily gifts.

I have often wondered about the unique circumstances surrounding Sharon's birth. Was Jean truly in labor, or was the obstetrical resident mistaken and Jean was only experiencing unusual and painful false labor pains. I don't really know and I don't know that it is important, because Sharon's birth was truly a miracle, as is each and every birth of any child anywhere. Yes, the birth of a child, in which we parents cooperate with God's designs and become in a sense co-creators with Him, is one of the greatest events that can happen to any human being.

— 6 —

The Short Cut

It was on one of the summer visits North with Jean and the children to spend time with my folks that a significant event occurred that would prove to be a spiritual turning point in my life. Dad and Mom had been retired for some time, and they both were enjoying their "Golden Years" together. Like any grandparents, they loved seeing the grandchildren.

The pediatric practice was doing well, and one of the advantages of an agreeable partnership was that I was able to take one or two weeks of vacation with the full knowledge that my patients were in the capable hands of my competent partner, Enrico Davoli.

My parents have always been deeply religious and faithful to the teachings of the Catholic Church. It was their love, good example and insistence on a Catholic school education that were primary factors in the development of my own religious faith. From the deepest recesses of my soul I came to believe in Jesus Christ as Our Lord and Saviour and in the Church He founded, the Roman Catholic Church, His Mystical Body here on earth.

His Church was the cornerstone of my spiritual and temporal life. However, in the wake of Vatican II and the dissent of many religious and laity from the authoritative teaching body of the Church, I found myself confused and floundering. In my search for the truth I started subscribing to theological journals and joining group discussions on current religious issues. I ended up more confused than ever.

It was on the occasion of this visit to my folks that I was spiritually rescued from all this bewilderment through a remarkable book.

Actually, I had been introduced to this book a number of years ago when my mother first told me about T*he Treatise of the True Devotion to the Blessed Mother* by Louis Marie Grignon De Montfort. The core of the book, written about the year 1700, revolves around a spiritual shortcut that St. Louis De Montfort recommended to be taken to the Heart of Jesus through an Act of Consecration of oneself to the Immaculate Heart of His Mother, Mary. The end result, of course, of this "shortcut" is an intensified spiritual life and liberation from confusion.

In this book, St. Louis recommends that the candidate planning to make this Act of Consecration set aside a period of thirty-three days of preparatory prayer, at the end of which he should "go to Confession and to Communion with the intention of giving (himself/herself) to Jesus Christ in the quality of a slave of love, by the hands of Mary." The essential part of the formula of consecration recommended by St. De Montfort reads as follows: "I (name), a faithless sinner, renew and ratify today in thy hands, O Immaculate Mother, the vows of my Baptism. I renounce forever Satan, his pomps and works; and I give myself entirely to Jesus Christ, the Incarnate Wisdom, to carry my cross after Him all the days of my life, and to be more faithful to Him than I have ever been before. In the presence of all the heavenly court I choose thee this day for my Mother and mistress. I deliver and consecrate to thee as thy slave, my body and soul, my goods, both interior and exterior, and even the value of all my good actions, past, present and future; leaving to thee the entire and full right of disposing of me, and all that belongs to me without exception, according to thy good pleasure, for the greater glory of God, in time and in eternity."

My father had recently made this Act of Consecration to the Blessed Mother using the devotional formula of St. Louis De Montfort, so now both he and my mother were encouraging me to consider taking the same spiritual step. I had casually read the Act of Consecration prayer in the past, but there were always a few things holding me back. The first obstacle was the word "slavery." To me it always had a demeaning connotation, one which made me feel uncomfortable. I didn't want to be anybody's "slave," even God's. The other stumbling block was that I thought this method would require a different way of relating to Jesus. I thought that I would no longer be able to go directly to Jesus in prayer, but would have to deliver, so to speak, my prayer to the Blessed Mother, who then would present it to Our Lord. It all seemed so complicated.

On either the second or third morning of this visit, I made these mental reservations known to my mother and father. I recall my mother handing me St. Louis's book, which I had never really read, and saying, "Why don't you make a deeper study of it, Joe, while you're here, and see what happens. By the way, I'm meeting with my Rosary group this evening; why don't you join us."

The remainder of this same day was a relaxing one spent with Jean and the children at the shore. I was able to read, despite interruptions, the first fifty pages or so. Still, I was not convinced. But at least I had a better idea of the meaning behind the Consecration which, once made, was meant to lead the candidate to recommit his life to Christ — but now through Mary, in Mary, with Mary and for Mary. In other words, just as she lived to do God's will, the candidate, now a spiritual copy of Mary, lives to do God's will.

That evening, after an enjoyable dinner with Mom, Dad, Jean and the children, I left with my mother for her Rosary group. I had taken along the book and had it with me during the Rosary recitation. It was during a period of meditation following the Rosary that I absent-mindedly opened the book and my eyes fell on the following passage: "Since for love of Mary we reduce ourselves freely to slavery, she, out of gratitude, will dilute our heart, intensify our love, and cause us to walk with giant steps in the way of God's Commandments. She delivers the soul from weariness, sadness, and scruples." These words stirred my heart and suddenly created in me a burning desire to consecrate myself to the Immaculate Heart of Mary. All previous doubts vanished, and I knew this was what I wanted to do. This sudden change was startling, and I could only attribute it to an increase in God's grace, to which I freely and immediately responded.

When we returned to the metropolitan area, I was determined to strictly follow St. Louis' preparatory method. I decided to make my Act of Consecration on the feast of the Immaculate Heart of Mary, which was approximately at the end of the preparatory period.

In his book, St. Louis suggests that the 33-day preparatory time be used as follows: an initial period of twelve days, during which I was encouraged to free myself from "the spirit of the world," was followed by a second period of three weeks. During the first week I was advised to humbly employ all prayers and pious actions in asking for a knowledge of myself and sorrow for my sins. The second week was to be devoted to acquiring an increased knowledge of the Blessed Virgin, and the third week was to be used in "the study of Jesus Christ."

I took this preparatory period very seriously and not only followed the daily prayer suggested by St. Louis, but also fasted and went to Mass daily. Ultimately, the day of my personal consecration arrived. It was the feast of the Immaculate Heart of Mary, and I dressed up in my best suit as if going to a feast. There were only six or seven people in church. Two elderly ladies sat in front of me and a few men and one younger woman were across the aisle. I noticed an arrangement of attractive flowers on the altar and wondered what they were there for. I recall that all during Mass my heart was both singing and experiencing a profound peace. I was very involved in the Mass and felt in a special way Our Lord's presence. It was my plan to make my act of consecration immediately following Holy Communion. Suddenly, about the time of the offertory, I noticed a faint, sweet odor much like that which might come from a bouquet of roses coming from the altar. I thought to myself how pleasant it was and that it must be coming from the flowers on the altar. I noticed, as Mass progressed, that the odor became more noticeable and at the time of the Consecration it was overpowering. After the Consecration it gradually decreased, and by the time I had received Communion, it had ceased altogether. After Communion, as planned, I silently made my Act of Consecration very slowly and solemnly. It was a wonderful moment, one which I shall eternally treasure.

When Mass was completed I remained until all the parishioners had left; I thought to myself that I had to examine those flowers more closely. Entering the Sanctuary, I approached the altar and realized the flowers were an arrangement of fall flowers, mostly a variety called mums. There were no roses at all in the arrangement. At first I was completely baffled, because by smelling the flowers I came to realize that they were completely odorless. It was only afterwards, upon reflection, that I realized the Blessed Mother, pleased with my Act of Consecration, had won for me this consolation from Jesus through His Mother.

For a brief moment a sinner like myself was permitted to understand more deeply what St. Paul said to the Ephesians when he stated, "He gave himself for us as an offering to God, a gift of pleasing fragrance." (Eph. 5:2).

This "pleasing fragrance" is offered up to the Father by the priest on our behalf every moment somewhere in the world. Praise God for His goodness.

The previous obstacles to my consecration proved to be nothing more than cardboard giants. When you ponder the meaning of the word "slavery," what does it really mean but the complete surrender of one's will to another. After all, isn't this what Christ did while on earth? He completely surrendered His Will to His Father's Will. This surrender reached a totality in the Garden of Gethsemane when Our Saviour did not shrink back from Calvary, but uttered His prayer of total abandonment, "Not My Will but Thy Will be done." The Blessed Mother, when the angel Gabriel announced to her that she was going to be the Mother of God, likewise totally surrendered her will to God's with her "Fiat," when she said, "Let it be done unto me according to thy word." Who was I to say I didn't want to be anybody's slave — not even God's!

And as far as Mary being an obstacle in my prayer relationship with her Son, Jesus, it was a ridiculous thought. After all, now all my prayers would pass to Jesus through Mary's hands. She being the good Mother she is, she would first perfume them, then bedeck them with flowers, and only then present my prayer to her Son. I felt any prayer she touched would be far more pleasing to God than my own, no matter how well-intentioned.

My understanding of this "short cut" to Our Lord's Heart has deepened over the years and has increased in me the desire to be more humble, to be more abandoned to God's Will and to be more inflamed with the desire to lead souls, through Mary, to Him. Jesus said, "Unless you become as little children you shall not enter the kingdom of Heaven." St. Louis's "short cut" permits easy access to spiritual childhood.

Imagine my joy many years later while paging through a Queens publication by the De Montfort Fathers when my eye fell on an article entitled, "Turning Point in My Life." It was an article that was an excerpt from Pope John Paul II's book, *Do Not Be Afraid* in which he says, in referring to his own Act of Consecration using the method of St. Louis De Montfort that, "reading this book was to be a turning point in my life....Whereas I had formerly held back, lest my Marian devotion should detract me from that due to Christ, I understood in the light of reading the treatise of Grignon De Montfort, that the very opposite was the case....It is, therefore, not a question of the one preventing us from seeing the other. Quite the contrary...it can be said that Christ Himself points out His Mother to the one who tries to know and love Him as He did to St. John at the foot of the Cross."

Since my Act of Consecration, I have been faithful within the limits of human frailty to its ideals. Daily Mass, meditation and prayer, particularly that humble prayer, the Rosary, and frequent use of the Sacrament of Reconciliation have kept me close to the Lord and His Mother.

In a hidden way, my newfound "short cut" affects my entire life, my relationship with my family, my patients, my partner, my friends and all others Our Lord sends my way.

— 7 —

New Year's Eve

I try to make it a habit each week to make a special visit to Church, with the specific intention of lighting a candle and praying to the Divine Physician for His aid and counsel in treating the children under my medical care. I can truthfully say in moments of crisis the Lord has never failed me.

I recall one night that with the able assistance of my wife and my own quick actions, a harrowing medical emergency was brought to a safe conclusion.

Jean and I were at a New Year's Eve party when the telephone call came. I was on duty and did not plan on the traditional champagne drink. This was a wise decision, for I would need all my wits this fateful evening.

Reluctantly, I dialed the number and listened to only one ring before someone quickly answered.

"Dr. Evers, Mr. Bishop here."

I sensed urgency in his voice.

"My boy David is very ill."

I couldn't for the life of me recall Mr. Bishop, but my memory for names has always been poor.

"Why, what seems to be wrong with him?"

"He's complaining about severe pain in his left hip joint; he has a fever and can't move his leg. I know it must be hurting him because he's the type of kid that hardly ever complains."

As he spoke, thoughts of septic arthritis and rheumatic fever flashed through my mind.

"Can you see anything unusual, Mr. Bishop?"

"Yes, it's awful red around the hip area."

"Mr. Bishop, let me see David in the office; let's say in thirty minutes."

Jean accompanied me, and apologizing to our hosts, we left.

As we pulled into the vacant parking lot surrounding the new building into which my partner and I had recently moved, we saw Mr. Bishop and his nine-year-old son waiting. Overhead, small, dark clouds paraded past a gibbous moon, tracing ghostly shadows on the concrete walls of the medical building. It gave an eerie cast to the otherwise peaceful evening.

I held the door open to the medical building as Mr. Bishop anxiously and hurriedly carried his son inside. I caught a fleeting glimpse of David's face as they passed through the door. He was a good-looking kid, but big-boned and gangly like his dad.

Seeing him prompted a recall of his last visit to my office. In particular I remembered his awkwardness in trying to negotiate the climb onto my three-foot examining table. Some boys leap onto the table with the nimbleness of Nijinsky executing a jete; others, like David, scale it as if it were Mt. Everest itself.

Tonight David was too ill to consider even that. His father carefully laid him on the table. I unbuckled his belt and exposed the site of infection. A nasty area of cellulitis, about eight inches in diameter, sprang into sight. His face, flushed with fever and distorted with pain, betrayed toxicity and bacterial infection. He squeezed his dad's hand tightly as I gently palpated the area.

"Does this hurt, David?" My fingers pressed two bulging lymph nodes in the upper portion of his leg.

"Yes, stop it."

A few tears immediately appeared in the nasal corner of each eye as David grimaced with pain. His father's large, powerfully built body hovered over his son like a protective shield, while his eyes surveyed my every move.

"Is it serious, Doc?"

"He's pretty sick, Mr. Bishop, but nothing so bad that a shot of penicillin won't take care of it."

Then what must have seemed like an afterthought to the father, I added, "He's not allergic to it, is he?"

"No, he's had it before and has never had any trouble with it."

David, overhearing this dialogue, started to whimper.

"Dad, do I have to get a shot?"

"Son, if it's going to help you get better, it's going to have to be done."

He gave David's left shoulder a fatherly squeeze as he spoke. David persisted, "But Dad, I don't want a shot. It's going to hurt."

With a note of impatience and embarrassment, his dad replied, "I know you don't, son, but you must be brave."

While Mr. Bishop attempted to both persuade and placate David, I prepared the injection. Six hundred thousand units should be enough, I thought to myself.

Holding the 10 cc vial of penicillin in my left hand, I disinfected the top of it with alcohol and jabbed the needled syringe into it.

"OK, David, roll over; this will be over in a second. I promise."

Very reluctantly he obliged. Holding the loaded syringe in my right hand, with a quick flick of my wrist I popped the needle into the right upper quadrant of his buttock. Drawing back on the syringe to make sure I wasn't in a blood vessel, I quickly rammed it home. A short yell from David, and it was all over.

"That should do it, Mr. Bishop; I'll write you out a prescription for the remainder of the penicillin that I want him to take."

Then nudging David, I asked, "Pills or liquid?"

David, still somewhat upset and angry over the whole affair, replied, "Liquid."

"Oh, yes, it's a bad enough infection that I'll want to see him tomorrow afternoon; right now, however, what I would like you to do is wait in the waiting room for about twenty to thirty minutes. My wife, a nurse, will be keeping an eye on David in case there is any kind of reaction."

"OK Doc, whatever you say."

Mr. Bishop picked his son up, went out to the waiting room and sat down with David on his lap. Jean sat down beside them.

I, in the meantime, started writing notes in David's medical chart.

No more than five minutes could have elapsed when Jean, the most non-hysterical person I've ever known, suddenly shouted, "Joe, hurry, David has just fainted."

Rushing into the waiting room, I knew instinctively what the problem was. David, his face ashen white, was slumped against his father's shoulder. The sight of David in profound anaphylactic shock secondary to the penicillin injection is a moment I'll never forget.

"Hurry, Mr. Bishop, bring David back into the examining room!"

Not fully aware of what was wrong with his son, yet detecting the sense of urgency in my voice, he asked, "What's wrong, Doc?"

I shot back the reply, "He's having a penicillin reaction."

By now we were inside the examining room. As Mr. Bishop laid his son on the table, I grabbed his right wrist, hoping against hope that I could detect a pulse. I could detect none.

"He's going to be OK, isn't he, Doc?"

I was unable to answer Mr. Bishop's question. The situation was critical. Saliva was frothing from David's mouth; his skin was blue-gray; and I knew that only a few minutes remained before irreversible brain could death ensue.

I was facing the moment every doctor dreads and which no doctor is completely equipped to handle.

Anaphylaxis — the word makes me shudder. The body is suddenly overwhelmed with a catastrophic drop in blood pressure due to an equally sudden release of a massive dose of a body chemical called histamine. A violent allergic reaction to an external foreign body substance such as penicillin or bee venom can trigger histamine release.

Like a tidal wave, the chemical floods the circulatory system, causing a total body relaxation of the small artery musculature, thus robbing the circulatory system of its peripheral resistance. Blood flow suddenly stagnates like swamp water. Without life-giving oxygen, body organs, like city lights late at night, start flicking off. The heart and brain are the first to go.

David's heart and brain were going.

My wife was by my side and in a very concerned yet calm voice said, "What do you want me to do?"

"One-half cc of adrenaline, fast."

Within seconds Jean had the syringe properly loaded and in my hand.

Ripping the boy's tee shirt off, I plunged the needle on the syringe like a dagger into his heart and quickly squirted in the life-giving fluid. With his blood flow all but stopped, the thought of giving it anywhere else didn't even enter my mind.

I heard Jean's voice call again.

"Shouldn't I call the ambulance?"

"Yes, by all means."

Withdrawing the needle, I bent over to start mouth to mouth resuscitation. Then I heard the most wonderful noise in the world. David groaned.

I looked at him and almost cried aloud. Pink flesh blossomed. Within seconds, his eyelids fluttered and as if nothing unusual had occurred, he said, "Dad, can we go home now?"

His father repeated his question of a few moments ago, even though it seemed like an hour.

"He's going to be OK, isn't he, Doc?"

"He's going to be fine, Mr. Bishop, he's going to be fine."

"Doc, Doc...can we help here?"

I had been concentrating so much on David's immediate problem that I had become divorced from the sights and the sounds of surrounding reality and was disoriented over the origin of this new voice. Looking over my shoulder to see who it was, I saw an ambulance driver and his first rider suddenly entering the room.

"I think the crisis is over, fellows." I explained to them the harrowing past few minutes. "I would like you to take him to Prince Edward's Hospital."

Placing David on their portable stretcher, they checked David's pulse and blood pressure and then started an IV infusion. Mr. Bishop never fully realized how close to death his son had come. I explained to him what a close call David had had and how it was necessary to admit him to the hospital.

Before going to bed that evening, my thanksgiving prayer to the "Divine Physician" was longer than usual, and I was sure that somewhere David's mother and father were joining me in this prayer.

David had to stay less than two days in the hospital, and except for a partial collapse of his left lung caused by the adrenaline needle, he was fine. A chest X-ray taken one week later revealed that the lung had completely re-expanded.

I promised myself that in the future I would give far fewer penicillin shots in the office. Only if the patient was vomiting and therefore unable to take penicillin by mouth would I give an injection. Penicillin remains the most important and frequently used antibiotic in our practice. It's just that now I administer it almost always by the oral route.

With Stethoscope and Scapular

— 8 —

Malpractice

It was just another telephone call to add to the confusion of a rapidly deteriorating Monday morning. First the air conditioner's condenser had frozen up for the umpteenth time and the office examining room, waiting rooms and laboratory were heating up like steam baths at the local Sahara Club.

For the fourth day in a row, Concetta, the new receptionist whom I had highly recommended to my colleague, had added the previous day's receipts incorrectly. Now she was having difficulty unlocking the strongbox which was needed to make change for the day.

Not surprisingly, my mind was elsewhere when Susan, our reliable nurse of many years, interrupted me in the midst of a six-month-old's physical to say that a rather demanding chap by the name of White wished to speak to me immediately on the phone.

I escaped to our hall phone, picked up the receiver and identified myself. Mr. White replied, "Dr. Evers, my name is John White. My wife and I are the couple who six weeks ago adopted a little boy whom you examined when a newborn at Prince Albert Hospital. Tell me, do you recall whether he had a heart murmur?"

I tried to recall who the infant was, and for the moment I couldn't. I vaguely recalled examining a baby who had been delivered by our local obstetrician and who was being placed for adoption. The health of the infant was to be verified by a pediatrician, in this case me, and if found to be normal, the baby was to be taken from the hospital by the adoptive parents. The customary manner of handling an adoption is through an adoption agency. This, however, was to be a direct placement from the mother to the prospective adoptive parents with neither party coming in contact with the other. The arrangements were orchestrated by a local lawyer and were perfectly legal.

"Mr. White," I replied, "I believe I do recall the infant in question, and no, I do not recall hearing a pathological heart murmur." I added as an afterthought, "Is there any problem?"

"Yes, there is, Doctor. The baby is now on the surgical service at Prince Albert Hospital. The doctors told us that the baby has a stomach tumor and a serious heart condition. Naturally, Mrs. White and I are quite concerned."

"I'm sorry to hear about the baby's problems, Mr. White, but if it is any comfort to you and your wife, the baby was in perfect health when I examined him."

That was the gist of my telephone conversation with Mr. and Mrs. White, and I dismissed the incident from my mind. As I returned to the six-month-old's physical, I was sorry to hear about the White's adoptive baby and was thankful that I didn't have to give this parent any bad news about a heart condition.

Several months later, on my first day back in the office following a delightful one-week vacation with my family in Panama City, Florida, I was greeted by my partner with the ominous words, "Joe, I think we have a problem."

I experienced simultaneously a chill and a generalized weakness. "We have a problem" is something I had never heard Enrico say. I have always admired his calmness, tranquillity and control in desperate situations. "Mr. Cool" is his trademark.

Well do I remember "Mr. Cool" in action one sticky, hot Friday afternoon not too long ago. Jeffery Lamb, age six, decided after getting his allergy shot that instead of wasting time sitting around the waiting room he would take his younger, four-year-old brother for an elevator ride. While their mother was engrossed in one of our waiting room's magazines, her young pioneers were playing "Up and Down the Elevator."

Unfortunately, the elevator jammed between floors. The boys, much to their credit, pushed the alarm button and the bell inside the elevator started clanging. The noise was deafening and the boys, justifiably terrified, started whooping and hollering at the top of their lungs. Meanwhile, Mrs. Lamb awakened from her literary escape, posted herself outside the elevator door and started shouting to the boys, "Mommy's right here — stay calm! Help is on the way."

The whole office was vibrating. The combination of the clanging bell, shouting mother and screaming elevator-captives made me feel as if I were enclosed in a large tin can while a giant pounded on the top of it with a sledge hammer. Patients and parents kept asking, "What is the matter?" Susan, our nurse, tried to reassure parents and children in our waiting room that the situation wasn't as bad as it sounded.

A perfect scenario for Enrico. With aplomb befitting Mr. Iceman and armed with only a screwdriver, he approached the erupting ironclad monster, gently pushed the mother aside, and pried the elevator doors apart. The inside compartment was halfway between the first and second floors. Drawn by the clamor, several onlookers had assembled outside the elevator door. In no time at all, with my partner directing the rescue, the boys were lifted to safety and rushed, sobbing, into their mother's grateful arms.

As I said, my partner does not get upset easily, so when he said, "We have a problem," my esophagus quaked and I replied, "OK, give it to me quickly — what's the problem?"

"Joe, have you ever heard of a Mr. and Mrs. White?" Before I could answer he continued, "Well, they are suing me in a malpractice action for failing to properly diagnose a pyloric tumor and a congenital heart defect in the infant boy they adopted some four months ago." There was a very long pause before he concluded, "Joe, I never heard of these people, and I never examined their baby."

"Yes, I know. It's not you they're suing, it's me. I saw that baby several months ago, and I'm sure he was in perfect health when I examined him."

By this time I was sweating. The mere mention of the word "malpractice" is enough to send chills up and down the spine of any doctor. My competence as a physician was being attacked, and the suggestion that I might actually be responsible for doing harm to a patient because of some careless action or oversight bothered me considerably.

"Joe, I have to admit it shook me up a bit," said Enrico. "I called our malpractice insurance agent the day I received the summons. I'm glad you weren't here."

"Why, what happened?"

"About four days after you and your family left for Florida, I think it was a Wednesday _ yeah, yeah, I know it was a Wednesday — I remember because that's one of the days Concetta works. By the way, Joe, she is having difficulty with her addition; we must talk to her and see if we can help her. Well, anyway, I was examining a little girl in one of the rooms when Concetta knocked on the door. Opening it, she informed me that a sheriff was in the waiting room and wanted to see me right away. She added that he was waving some papers in his hand. I mumbled some excuse to the mother of the patient I was examining, stepped into the hall and there, bearing down on me like an 18-wheeler, was this overweight, red-faced sheriff, shouting, 'Dr. Davoli, this is a summons for you to appear in court to answer malpractice charges placed by the plaintiff, Mr. and Mrs. John White.'"

Enrico took a deep breath and with a suffering stare said, "Joe, you know we've never been sued and I felt completely bewildered standing eyeball to eyeball in our hall with this very intense sheriff waving those papers in my face."

Knowing I was the intended victim of those papers instead of my unfortunate partner, I asked, "What did you do?"

"What could I do? I accepted the summons, and then Concetta ushered him out."

"Enrico, I'm sorry you had to go through that, but don't forget that we don't have a problem, only I have a problem. Once the lawyer checks the hospital chart and finds only my name on it, then your worries will be over. I'm sure I'll be hearing from somebody soon."

During the ensuing days, I reviewed the case a thousand times. I started wondering if I had missed an abnormal heart sound, but knew I would have to be deaf to do that. Subconsciously, I kept looking over my shoulder for a fat, red-faced sheriff with the ominous summons in his hand.

Days dragged into weeks, weeks into months; still no sheriff, no call from anyone. I started wondering if my partner had imagined the whole affair or if the plaintiffs had either forgotten the case or had decided to drop it.

Malpractice cases aren't that simple; no one forgets; it's just that the law — although relentless — proceeds very slowly.

Our insurance company least of all did not forget and had assigned our case to one of their lawyers. Thus one bright and sunny morning, Enrico and I met with the attorney in a small sound-proof room in the library at County General Hospital to give a deposition. As the three if us sat around a small table the attorney introduced himself. "Doctors, my name is Jim Larkin, and I will be handling your case." He placed a large black briefcase on the table, opened it, and pulled out a recording device. Reminding us we were under oath, he flicked on a switch and started to question us.

"Dr. Davoli, as you know, the parents of the adopted baby are suing you because of your alleged failure to diagnose a heart condition and a stomach tumor."

I interrupted, "Correction, Mr. Larkin. I don't know why they are suing Dr. Davoli, because I'm the only one who was involved with the infant."

"I don't know, either, Dr. Evers, but we will leave that to their lawyer to straighten out, because as the case stands now, they indeed are suing the wrong doctor." With a half-smile on his face and executing a self-satisfied upward thrust of his eyebrows, he continued.

"Let me ask you, Dr. Evers, did you hear anything in your examination of the baby's heart that would lead you to believe the baby had a heart problem?"

"No, Mr. Larkin, the heart sounded normal to me; I heard no pathological heart sound."

"What is the difference between a pathological and a non-pathological heart sound?"

"It is a degree of loudness or intensity; the pathological heart sound is, as a rule, much louder than the non-pathological or innocent heart sound, or murmur, as it is sometimes called."

"I see, thank you. Let me continue. The plaintiffs are also accusing you of failing to diagnose a stomach tumor for which the infant had to undergo an operation for repair at eight weeks of age. Could you enlighten me as to what they are referring to?" His half-smile had disappeared and his now motionless face unnerved me.

"Certainly, Mr. Larkin. A condition called pyloric tumor or pyloric stenosis is not a cancerous tumor at all; rather, it's an abnormal enlargement of muscle fiber around the terminal end of the stomach where it empties into the intestine. A baby begins to develop symptoms of recurrent projectile vomiting at about three to six weeks of age. It is not diagnosable at birth, only at the time of symptom development."

Mr. Larkin seemed nonplused by my response, merely blinked a few times and cryptically asked, "How is the diagnosis made?"

"By palpating the baby's stomach. About half the time, a large marble-like lump can be felt. However, an X-ray of the stomach with a barium swallow is the only way of making the diagnosis."

Enrico interrupted, "It's all so absurd, Mr. Larkin. The diagnosis is impossible before three to four weeks of age unless the doctor is gifted with X-ray vision."

Larkin, an intelligent man, immediately replied, "Wait a minute, wouldn't it be possible to feel the tumor at birth if in half the cases you can feel it three weeks later?"

"Not really," my partner replied. "Rarely, if ever, can it be felt at birth. The tumor just isn't large enough. During the succeeding weeks it enlarges as the muscle tries to push food through the narrow opening into the stomach."

I threw my hands up in a gesture of disbelief. "They have no case on these two accusations, Mr. Larkin. I heard no abnormal murmur, nor was it possible to diagnose a pyloric tumor at the time I examined the baby."

"Thank you, Doctors. It seems obvious from what you have said here that there is no substance to the Whites' complaint."

Mr. Larkin moved the switch of the recorder to the "off" position, unceremoniously concluding the interview. Almost as an afterthought, he blankly stated, "By the way, you know they didn't adopt the baby."

Enrico and I looked at each other in amazement.

"Who wants a kid with problems," I sarcastically said.

Enrico added, "Well, maybe the reason for not adopting the baby is that they couldn't handle all the extra expense it would demand, or they felt inadequate."

I hadn't thought of that and felt ashamed of my judgmental remark.

Several months passed, and I had successfully buried the whole affair in a forgotten area of my brain when the malpractice insurance lawyer called to inform me that the plaintiffs were proceeding with the suit, that their lawyer had discovered that it was I, not my partner, who was the defendant and a calendar date for the trial had been set four months hence. I was not terribly surprised by his call, and despite my confidence in being vindicated, the fact that I was going to have to appear in court bothered me.

It was a gloomy, cloudy day and so were my spirits when later that day I almost collided with Charlie as he exited from the medical building elevator. I have known Charlie for eighteen years. He is an excelled internist, an astute diagnostician and a true friend, but he does have a few failings — most notable of which are his complete and total honesty and his tendency to look on the pessimistic side of some issues. We struck up a conversation and, looking for solace, I mentioned the case.

"You can't imagine what it's like, Charlie. Even though I know I've done my best, even though I'm sure no malpractice exists, I keep thinking that some smart prosecuting lawyer might come up with something that will end up with me losing the suit."

There was a long pause before Charlie answered. He didn't look directly at me, but gazed over my right shoulder and appeared to be deep in thought.

"Now wait a minute, Joe, let's see if I have this straight."

I was used to Charlie's ponderous replies. I've always held him in awe. He graduated cum laude from Jefferson School of Medicine and is a member of Cerebral, an intellectual club whose entrance card is an IQ. in the range of 150 or so.

"You say you're being sued because you allegedly missed hearing an obvious heart murmur and failed to diagnose a pyloric tumor. I thought it was not possible to pick up a pyloric tumor until three to four weeks of life, and then it required an operation to repair the obstruction."

"Correct, Charlie. The baby was operated on at Prince Albert Hospital and, just prior to surgery, the heart problem was detected. When the adoptive parents found out that the baby had a heart problem in addition to the pyloric tumor, they refused to continue with permanent adoption."

Charlie's mouth hung open in disbelief. "What? Why would they do that?"

"I'm not sure; there could be a number of reasons. Perhaps they figured it would be too much expense for them to handle, or they felt they couldn't cope with a handicapped child."

"But why are they suing you if they don't intend to adopt the child?"

"The usual — pain and suffering, and also for the reimbursement of the hospital expenses for the pyloric tumor operation. They have no way of nailing me on the pyloric tumor. Any good lawyer should be able to clear me on that. However, I don't know what's going to happen about the heart problem."

"Can it be diagnosed at the time of birth, Joe?"

"Sometimes yes; sometimes no. All I know is that I did not hear any loud murmur on this little baby when I examined him in the hospital nursery twelve hours after birth. I believe I may have heard a soft, innocent murmur of the ductus arteriosus before it closed, but I can't swear to it, and I didn't mark it down on the chart. In fact, all I indicated was that the heart was normal."

Charlie paused and thought for a few moments. "Let's see if I remember my pediatrics. The ductus arteriosus, isn't that the blood vessel that's responsible for delivering oxygen-rich blood to the baby while it's still inside the mother's uterus?"

"Right."

"And doesn't it close shortly after birth?"

"Very good, Charles, usually within the first twenty-four hours."

"I see, Joe; then the whole case rests on the intensity or loudness of the murmur?"

"That's about right, Charlie, and I can say that I didn't hear any loud pathological murmur."

This is when old honest Charlie hit me with a sledgehammer. "Joe, I don't mean to worry you, but have you had your hearing checked lately?"

My eyes opened wide, and I blankly stared at him, dumbfounded by his query.

"I hate to say this, but there are times when I wonder if you don't have a hearing problem."

"Hey, Charlie, you're crazy. I'm sure there's nothing wrong with my hearing."

"Well, Joe, you're probably right, but any good lawyer who suspected a hearing deficiency and who was smart enough might hang you on it if indeed you do have a problem."

The conversation drifted to other matters and when we parted company my spirits were lower than ever. Perhaps Charlie was right. From time to time my family had mentioned they thought something was wrong with my hearing. My father has had a definite hearing loss, and maybe I had inherited it. I started perspiring just thinking about the possibility. What if I did miss a pathological murmur. Perhaps I should have my hearing checked.

Three months passed before I heard from the lawyer again. He informed me that the case was set for a court hearing in one month.

"By the way, Dr. Evers, nothing's changed, has it? You are still pleading innocent..."

I silently groaned inside and felt a sweaty palm grasping the telephone receiver. My appointment with Irv Goldstein's otology nurse for a hearing test was set for the end of the week. Summoning up all the positive thinking I could muster, I croaked, "Of course."

It was a Friday afternoon, and compulsive as I am I was there on the stroke of 2:00 PM for my scheduled appointment. I was not in the best frame of mind, and the autologist annoyed me practically the moment I stepped inside the door.

"Right in here, Doctor, eh... What is your name again?"

"Evers."

"Evers, well fine, if you will please follow me this way."

She escorted me into the small coffin-like chamber that served as an auditory examining room. Following her instructions, I placed a pair of earphones over my ears. The room, lined with noise-absorbent tile, was completely enclosed except for a small window. With a vacant smile, she peered at me through the small window. Feeling as if I were a prisoner, I waited for my observer's next move.

"Doctor," her voice through the loudspeaker startled me, "raise your right hand when you hear a noise in your right ear and your left hand when you hear a noise in your left ear."

I had the distinct impression she was bored by the whole affair. "OK," I replied, "any time you're ready."

"Sorry, I can't hear you," she sweetly cooed.

"You mean the loudspeaker only works one way?" I shouted.

"Sorry, I can't hear you," she purred once again.

I wondered if this woman knew what she was doing.

"Shall we proceed, Doctor, eh" she fumbled through my chart looking for my name, "Evers?"

I felt as though I were strapped in a miniature electric chair, with a smiling executioner leering at me. The only thing missing was the row of newspaper reporters.

"Yeah, turn on the juice, I want it to be over with as quickly as possible," I yelled.

"Sorry, I can't hear you," she replied.

I said nothing; I just kept mouthing the word, "Start, start." If there were any more delays, I feared I would melt from frustration and heat exhaustion.

It was forever, it seemed, before I heard the first "BEEP," and I shot my hand up into the air. A few moments passed..."BEEP," and I shot my other hand up. She nodded approvingly and smiled her sweetest smile. There was a long pause before I heard anything more. Suddenly her sweet smile disappeared and she quizzically looked at me. Thoughts started to tumble through my mind. Was she pushing her beeper button and I wasn't picking it up? What if I flunked this darn test? A good attorney would make Saturday morning hash out of me.

I could just hear the attorney, "Doctor, you say you heard no abnormal heart sound, is that correct?"

"Well..."

"Please answer yes or no, Doctor."

"No."

"And, Doctor, have you recently taken a hearing test? Remember, you're under oath, Doctor. Please answer yes or no."

"Yes."

"And what did the hearing test reveal? Oh! By the way, it appears you and I have the same ear, nose and throat specialist."

"BEEP!" My fantasy was interrupted. I shot my left hand up; "BEEP," and I shot my right hand up. I noticed that the quizzical look had disappeared and she was smiling; in fact, her smile was getting brighter and brighter. Suddenly all was quiet, and I knew in my bones the test was over. Drenched with perspiration and immobile with fear, I awaited the verdict. The door opened and, like an angel, the woman rang out with the words, "Dr. Evers, your hearing is perfect." It was better than a commuted sentence; it was a governor's pardon. If I could have tap danced, I would have.

I made a mental note as I left the office to tell Irv what a competent, beautiful, loving nurse he had performing the audiometry testing.

Two days before the scheduled trial, Jim Larkin called. "Dr. Evers, are you sitting down?"

"Yes — why?"

"Well, you'll never believe what's happened. The Whites are dropping the malpractice suit."

"You're kidding me!"

"No, no, I'm serious. Apparently sometime within the last month, according to the Whites' attorney, the couple made a marriage encounter weekend. Obviously something happened to make them change their minds. I don't know the details, but you can forget the whole affair."

I was delighted over the news, but puzzled as to what had occurred to change the Whites' minds. It must have been about a week later when a letter arrived at the office, which read:

Dear Doctors,

My wife and I would like to apologize and ask your forgiveness for the anxiety and difficulty we have caused you because of our malpractice suit against you.

You may wonder about our change of heart; well, it was all the Lord's doing. My wife and I just finished making a marriage encounter weekend and after much discussion, thought and prayer we were brought to realize how selfish we were in not accepting the baby and now know that if any baby needs the love and care of parents it is a handicapped baby.

Furthermore, in talking with parents who take their children to you we have discovered what a competent and caring physician you are and we had no right in assuming anything else.

The baby has been with a foster family since we gave him up. Please pray for us, because we are going to talk with the agency again and see if we can have our son back.

Sincerely,

Mr. and Mrs. John White

It was about two months after the case was dropped that I was looking at the appointment book and asked, "Concetta, I notice a new family is coming in next week by the name of White, and they are bringing in their eighteen-month-old son, John. Do you know anything more about them?"

"I can't remember much, Dr. Evers, except that they told me that although neither of you had ever met, you both would have much to discuss."

"Hmmm, I wonder — thank you, Concetta, and but the way — how is that pocket calculator working out?"

"Well, have you noticed any mistakes in the daily log?"

"Say no more, Concetta, say no more."

It was while at a weekend retreat a short time after the trial was dismissed that I was pondering over some of the spiritual lessons I had learned.

I often had heard the Gospel imperative, "Judge not and you shall not be judged," but yet how easy it had been for me both vocally and mentally to judge the Whites as unloving adoptive parents. Thoughts like, "They discarded that little baby from their life just like one would attempt to get rid of a car that was a lemon," or "How lucky that little baby was not to have them as parents" had paraded through my mind.

How very opposite is my partner Henry who, yielding to the action of the Spirit, not only remains "cool" in hectic situations, but also does his best not to make critical remarks — or at the most will blame an imperfection or failing in a person on ignorance or infirmity.

While reading through the beautiful spiritual guide, Introduction to the Devout Life by St. Francis de Sales, I am reminded by the Saint to "never pass judgment on our neighbor."

I concluded this retreat with the firm resolution, through God's grace, of putting this command into action.

— 9 —

Housecall

The shrill cry of the phone split the night, jolting me upright in bed. The dial of the clock faintly glowed 3:00 a.m. I fumbled for the receiver. The sensation is always the same — twenty years in practice and the old bones have never accepted Alexander Graham Bell's fiendish invention. My heart races. I fumble for the phone, and find myself muttering, "This can't be happening to me." Ben Casey, maybe; Marcus Welby, certainly — but why me?

All the previous day, Enrico and I had been knee-deep with patients fighting the winter flu. The press had been loaded with scare stories that Swine flu was on the march and, like the four horsemen of the Apocalypse, the flu was about to devastate and devour all in its path. In actuality, a rather mild form of influenza had been rampaging for a week. The children were exhibiting the usual symptoms of cough, fever, and sore throat seen so commonly with this illness, but there was no cause for alarm. There was nothing to suggest the dreaded Swine flu. Needless to say, parents could not be expected to know this, and with the news media bombarding them with frightening predictions, they were bringing their little ones to the office in droves.

To say the least, I was exhausted from the sheer numbers and resentful over the telephone's heartless invasion of my sleep. As I held the receiver to my ear, the answering service informed me that Dr. Norman Fossedal wished to speak to me about his daughter, who was running a high fever.

I knew Norm well. His eighteen-month-old daughter, Sarah, had been under the care of my partner since birth. She is a beautiful, dark-haired little girl with dazzling ebony eyes and long, graceful, curving eyelashes. Her swarthy, bull-necked father is totally under her spell.

Unfortunately, Sarah has a congenital heart defect consisting of a moderate-sized hole in the ventricular septum, the large muscular wall that separates the major heart chambers. Occasionally a hole the size of Sarah's will cause problems, and indeed, recently she had developed signs of minimal heart failure and was placed on digitalis, a heart medication. Norm, a fourth-year medical student, is already a promising physician and a father.

I rubbed my eyes briskly as I waited for Norm to answer the phone. I had been told that brisk rubbing, like cold water in the face, helps to awaken one.

"Dr. Evers, please forgive me for calling you at this unearthly hour."

"That's okay, Norm. What's wrong?" His voice, usually relaxed, as is his demeanor, now sounded tense.

"Well, Sarah is running a 104-degree temperature, and I feel terribly guilty about it."

"Oh, why is that, Norm?"

"Well, a few days ago she was fussy, had a cold and was pulling at her ears. They looked a little red so I put her on some antibiotic."

"Sounds to me like perfectly acceptable treatment so far."

"What I feel bad about is that after she was acting well for a few days, I discontinued it. I suppose it was too soon."

"What do her ears look like now, Norm?"

"I'm not sure. I don't trust my judgment. Also, I'm just plain scared. Her heart's racing, her face is flushed and she's breathing very rapidly."

Poor Norm, I knew just how he felt. We fathers generally are poor physicians when it comes to diagnosing and treating members of our own family. We are either under or over concerned and our judgment is not the best.

In the calmest 3:00 AM voice I could muster, I replied, "Norm, we are in the midst of a December flu epidemic and chances are, it probably is nothing more than a virus."

There was a numbing silence on the other end of the line followed by a long sigh. "Perhaps I should take her to the emergency room," he replied.

I was sure from the symptoms he recited that the problem could be handled at home with fever control measures, and that the actual physical examination could be postponed until morning. On the other hand, if I suggested this, I knew that Norm would agree, but would remain uncomfortable. He hated to bother me, he hated to drag me out of bed at this hour, but at the same time he was terribly concerned about his daughter and just could not trust his own judgment.

"Norm, give me directions to your home, and I'll be right over."

"I really hate to do this to you, Doctor, but you'll never know how relieved I am that you are coming."

It was a cold, clear, December night. A light snow had fallen earlier that evening, spreading a blanket of crystalline white powder. Standing in the driveway and admiring the star-bedecked sky, I inhaled deeply the crisp night air. It reminded me of my childhood back in frigid Buffalo, New York, where it would have been a perfect night for ice-skating or night hockey. As I walked toward the car, I felt the ground crinkle under my feet.

Stretching my neck out the auto window, I carefully backed out of the driveway and thanked the glowing half moon for illuminating the semi-hidden drainage ditch to the right of the driveway entrance. A wheel ensnared in its grip would mean a delay of several hours.

While driving to Norm's home, I reflected that it was only a week ago that he spent an afternoon instructing me on the secrets of installing a valve cover gasket in my ailing '73 sedan.

Norm is a "Jack of all trades," with gifted hands. He is considering internal medicine as his future specialty, but I think surgery is where he actually belongs. He was very patient with me that day when we worked on my car, considering that he was dealing with a person with the automotive mentality of a kindergarten student. What's under the hood of an automobile has always been a mystery to me, and I have suffered for years from acute auto incompetency.

My physician's bag was next to me in the front passenger seat of the car, and as I drove I found myself patting it like a faithful pet. This bag, made of a high quality black leather, was Jean's first Christmas gift to me, and I've always loved it. Inside the bag is more than enough room for my stethoscope, blood pressure cuff and otoscope. Its countless little drawers and recessed compartments are perfect for storing syringes, medications, bandages and the like. There is even space for a box lunch. Although worn at the edges after twenty years of use, I carried it with pride as I entered Norm's apartment.

"What an hour to drag you out," exclaimed the smiling father, "but thanks a million for coming."

Judith, his slim, attractive wife, echoed her husband's apology.

"No problem, folks. Where's the little patient?"

"She's in the back room, Doctor," replied Judith. "Please, right this way."

I followed her down the short hallway, and I couldn't help but notice a beautiful picture of the Madonna with Child hanging at the end of the hall. There was something about the picture that made me think the artist must have been Spanish. Continuing on the heels of Sarah's mother, within moments I was at her bedside. Sarah gazed up at me from her little bed and apprehensively scrutinized me. Instantly she knew I wasn't Granddaddy or any other friendly face. She searched her memory bank, it registered, and I was discovered. She howled with fright, and I could almost hear her thinking, "Ah! there he is, that smiling abomination with long spidery fingers, who probes, pinches, and punches me in the stomach and then pries my mouth open with a gigantic wooden plank and plunges it inside my mouth. Meanwhile my mommy and daddy say, 'He's such a nice man Sarah. He's your friend, and he's going to make you well.'"

No wonder she screamed as I approached her. Could Count Dracula expect any other type of welcome? I tried all the tricks of the trade, the soothing voice, the gentle touch, the friendly smile, but it was a lost cause. I was finished before I started. She had seen too many doctors in her short life and was just plain terrified.

Sarah's mother, embarrassed with her daughter's behavior, gasped, "Doctor, how are you going to be able to tell anything with Sarah screaming and thrashing about like she is?"

"Don't worry, Judy," I said. "Twenty or so years in pediatrics has its rewards. I'll be able to obtain all the information I need."

I asked Judith to place Sarah on her lap. I then listened to her chest. She continued to flail her arms and protest.

"Oh, sweetheart, please calm down so the doctor can listen to you."

"Actually, Judy, she's telling us a lot. She can't be too ill to be so active, and for sure she can't be in heart failure."

Judy wistfully smiled as she continued to restrain her child and said, "Well, I really thank God for that."

I purposefully prolonged my examination of the lungs, hoping Sarah would calm down, but it was futile. She continued to howl, scratch and screech like a cornered cat. Despite all the fanfare, I was able to obtain the necessary information to diagnose the problem. Her heart, although pounding, was not excessively rapid and its rhythm was steady. When I felt her liver, which is located in the right upper portion of the abdomen, I was relieved, for it confirmed my impression that she was not in heart failure. Its edge was sharp and it was normal in size. If she were in heart failure, the edge would be blunted and the liver would be enlarged.

The high fever, the slight runny nose, now a river due to her crying and the mild red throat, all pointed to the viral flu syndrome with which my associate and I had been bombarded for the last few weeks.

"Norm, it's nothing more than the flu. She'll be feverish for a day or two, but no more."

I could identify with the welcome relief that he and Judith immediately experienced. Memories flashed through my own mind, the times when I was the father and not the doctor. There was the occasion when our youngest daughter, Tara, while playing with her older sister, fell full weight on her abdomen. I was convinced that her continued pain and pallor represented a possible ruptured spleen. Recklessly ripping out of our driveway, I thought I would never reach the emergency room. Then the seemingly endless wait for one of my surgical colleagues to examine our daughter. And finally the magic sentence: "Nothing to worry about, Joe. Just an injured muscle."

The concern, the anxiety, all evaporated. Having experienced this feeling first-hand, it is exhilarating to evoke and witness the same response from parents.

After prescribing some simple measures to Norm and Judith to relieve Sarah's symptoms, they invited me to join them in a 4:00 AM snack of coffee and cookies. The coffee with its priming pump, caffeine, can be a pediatrician's waterloo. No matter, the night was too far gone to consider sleep, anyway.

As I drove homeward through the stillness of the early morning, the snow-tinged trees and shrubbery emitted a sense of tranquility. The peacefulness of the moment and the success of the nocturnal visit made me think of the Spanish Madonna, and I couldn't help but recall the words of Our Lady of Guadalupe to the Indian convert Juan Diego, "Do not be troubled or disturbed about anything, do not fear illness, grievous happenings or pain. Are you not under my shadow, my protection."

— 10 —

The Rosary

The Rosary is my favorite prayer, and over the many years I have been promoting it, I have collected some interesting and humorous stories.

I recall the occasion a few years ago when Rory O'Sullivan, Ellen O'Sullivan's youngest, sent me a thank-you note. Quizzical as to its contents and knowing I would want to save both the letter and the envelope, I gently separated its adhesive edge with my fingers and removed the letter.

It was only three days ago, prior to receipt of the letter that I had made a house call to the large, white framed house. As I knocked on the front door, which was painted a brilliant red, I was amused at the warning on a small sign jutting from the ground: "TRESPASSERS WILL BE EATEN," and I wondered if the trespasser-eating creature considered me fair game and even now might be picking up my scent.

An attractive young woman, Mrs. O'Sullivan's maid I assumed, answered the door and ushered me inside.

"Good to see you, Doctor Evers, Mrs. O'Sullivan's been expecting you," and pointing in the direction she wanted me to head, she continued, "why don't you go right through that open door. The stairs are to your left. Just go right up them."

With a half-smile on her face, she hesitated a bit before adding, "Oh, by the way, be careful not to trip over the dog; he usually sleeps at the bottom of the stairs."

With caution I proceeded in the suggested direction and was not surprised to see a large black Irish Retriever stretched full length, sound asleep, on the bottom step, blocking my passage.

I knew Irish Retrievers were good bird dogs, and I wondered for a moment about their ability to flush out pediatricians. Would I be his main course, or just dessert. Hoping for the best, I leaped over him and bounded up the stairs. Old Irish, bless his heart, without so much as a nose twitch or tail swish, slept on.

Nearing the top of the stairs, I heard Mrs. O'Sullivan's voice, "Right up here, Doctor." Reaching the second floor, I turned to my left and was immediately greeted by Rory's mother. Over the years that I have had the privilege to render medical care to their younger children, I've always secretly enjoyed any encounter with them and their mother, whom I deeply admire and respect.

Shaking my hand and with obvious sincerity in her voice Mrs. O'Sullivan said, "It's so good of you to come, Doctor. Please follow me; Rory's right in the bedroom at the end of this hall." As I followed her toward the bedroom, I caught a glimpses of the many wall hung photographs of their family boasting eight children. Such happiness radiated from their smiles.

"In here, Doctor, don't trip over that rug," then reaching her daughter's bedside and placing her hand on her head, she exclaimed, "Oh the poor child, she is so terribly hot, and listen to that cough."

The cough, high-pitched and barking in nature, did sound bad. Only her head was visible; the rest of her body was covered by a blue blanket which bobbed up and down every time she coughed.

"Sit up, darling, so the doctor can examine you."

Rory, her blond hair in disarray, pushed herself to a sitting position. I could tell by how she moved how badly she must be feeling, but like most children she didn't complain.

After five minutes or so, I concluded my examination and reported to her mother that Rory's illness was nothing more than a croup virus. I recommended a cough expectorant and a decongestant and reached into my pocket for a prescription pad on which to write a few instructions. My fingers found my rosary instead of the pad. Recalling Mrs. O'Sullivan's deep devotion to the Rosary, I instinctively drew it from my pocket and held it before Rory's eyes and asked, "Rory, would you like this pretty blue Rosary?"

Rory, though subdued by her illness, managed a bright smile and answered, "Oh! yes, it's beautiful! Thank you so much." Rory's mother added, "That's so very kind of you, Doctor. Thank you."

I knew that she meant it, for on frequent occasions I have observed her at daily Mass in our local parish, approaching Holy Communion with her beads in her hand. The faith is very important to this good and gracious woman and has sustained her over the years in her own personal journey through this valley of sorrows.

As I held Rory's letter in my hand I was impressed by the carefully constructed penmanship and smile as I read:

Dear Doctor,

I would like to thank you for the beautiful blue Rosary you were so kind to give me. However, I must tell you that even though I am saying the prayers, I am still quite sick with my cold.

Sincerely,
Rory O'Sullivan

Oh dear, I thought. Little Rory in her innocence was expecting an immediate healing, or at least a more rapid one. I applauded her expectations, recalling Jesus' words that if we had the faith of a mustard seed, we could move mountains.

I take comfort in the common bond that the O'Sullivans and I share, our love for the Rosary. Our roots are the same — our families are Irish — and the Irish have always had a deep love for this prayer. However, it's more than my Irish heritage that is responsible for my devotion to the Rosary. Its attraction stems not only from my parents, but in a very particular way from my grandmother, Grandmother Evers. Evers is German and was her married name, but Colbert is very Irish and was her maiden name. She possessed this faith that Jesus referred to, this child-like faith that can move mountains.

And speaking of mountains, my grandmother was born at the foot of the Gaulty Mountains in County Cork, Ireland, and lived there until her early twenties. A determined and adventuresome young girl, she emigrated to the United States in the late 19th Century.

The story goes that she believed she had a vocation to become a nun, but on the voyage across the Atlantic she met a handsome and equally determined young man from Hamburg, Germany. He wooed her and won her heart, and she in turn accepted his proposal, on one condition: that he would forsake his own Protestant religion and convert to Catholicism. This he did. Grandmother had moved her first mountain.

They married, set up housekeeping in Boston, begot six children, adopted a seventh and had seventeen grandchildren. My father, the youngest of the six with the same wanderlust in his blood, married an Irish gal by the name of McCarthy, my mother, and migrated to Buffalo, New York. I was an infant at the time of this move.

My brother and sister were born in Buffalo, and each year our family of five would faithfully travel east to visit the grandparents in Boston.

These were joyous times, with many aunts and uncles to visit and a bundle of cousins to play with. Grandmother Evers, to this day, evokes special memories — memories of thick, tasty potato soup filing the bowl to the brim, lush blueberry pies, and her merry, merry inquiries as to my appetite, health, friends and school work. Richest of all memories, however, is the recollection of her seated in her favorite rocking chair tolling her beads.

Her face, arched by gossamer snow-white hair, was creased with the most pleasant, peaceful wrinkles I had ever seen. The glow in her eyes and the perpetual smile on her face were but a reflection of the Christian joy that reigned supreme in her heart.

Grandmother Evers loved the Rosary and had great faith in its power with the Almighty. Dad used to remind me, "You know Joe, your Nanna had six children and seventeen grandchildren, and the boys of both generations went through both World Wars without a scratch. She told me more than once she wasn't surprised; she was sure it was her faithfulness to the recitation of her daily Rosary that won God's protection for them all.

From childhood I have always cherished the Blessed Mother's promise of eternal life to the person who is faithful to the recitation of the daily Rosary.

This, of course, is only one of the promises to the Christian who piously recites the Rosary daily. Saint Louis De Montfort, in his famous book, *The Secret of the Rosary*, recorded all fifteen of the promises revealed by the Blessed Mother to Blessed Alan and Saint Dominic. There are two of the promises that are of particular comfort in today's difficult times. One is the promise that "whoever shall recite the Rosary devoutly, applying himself to the consideration of its sacred mysteries shall never be conquered by misfortune. God will not chastise him in His justice, he shall not perish by an unprovided death; if he be just he shall remain in the grace of God, and become worthy of eternal life." The second particularly attractive promise states, "All those who propagate the holy Rosary shall be aided by me in their necessities."

It is necessary while saying each decade to meditate on the fifteen different highlights in the life of Christ. The five Joyful Mysteries reflect the events surrounding His birth and childhood. The five Sorrowful Mysteries concentrate on His passion and death. The five Glorious mysteries draw our attention to His Resurrection, Ascension and events surrounding His Apostles and His Mother, Mary.

I was explaining the Rosary one day to about sixty fourth-grade school children. During the talk a little girl politely interrupted me and asked, "Doctor, why do you call the Bible stories about Jesus, the stories that we are supposed to think about, when we say the Rosary, mysteries?"

I told her quite honestly, I didn't know why and had often wondered about that myself.

Suddenly, a little fellow in the rear of the audience shot up his hand and I motioned to him to speak. "Doctor, I know why they are called mysteries." I answered that I would appreciate knowing why. He then responded, "Because, Doctor, we can never know enough about Jesus." I thought that was the best response I had ever heard on the subject.

It is praiseworthy when saying the Rosary not only to say the prayers with great devotion while meditating on the mysteries, but to pray for various personal intentions with the expectation of our intentions being heard and answered. The intentions can be many and varied — the cure of a sick husband, wife or child; the conversion of a spiritually lost friend; the reversal of financial misfortune, to name a few.

I have had great success in promoting all these aims of the Rosary through a variation of the Rosary, called the Living Rosary.

The modus operandi of the Living Rosary is a little different. It is a community-oriented prayer made up of five, ten or fifteen people. The ideal number is fifteen. Each person each day resolves to say one decade of the Rosary for the intentions of all the other members involved.

Each member receives from the team leader a Living Rosary Calendar and a list of intentions of the other members so as to know what decade to recite and meditate on and what intentions to pray for.

Through the power of the press, I have been able to generate interest in the Living Rosary in hundreds of parishes across the United States as well as in hundreds of mission posts abroad, particularly Africa and India. I estimate about 30,000 people are now using this prayer method and, judging from the responses I have received, it has been very effective.

One of my favorite Living Rosary spin-offs was the organization of the Living Rosary pen-pal team, whereby through the U.S. mail and prayer the elderly, the lonely, the ill and the infirm, are united with one other.

In an article I wrote for *The Family* magazine, published by the Daughters of St. Paul, in discussing the pen-pal teams, I said, "I received a beautiful letter just a few weeks ago from Dorothy, age 60, who lives in Michigan. She is a member of one of many pen-pal teams and is joined in prayer through the United States Mail with Mary in Maryland, who suffers with emphysema; Marie in New Jersey, who just recently lost her husband; Pat who lives in Michigan and who has personal problems; and finally, Clara who lives in New York and suffers with diabetes. What cheers my heart is that she states, "We are doing fine; two of us have reaped our intentions through the Living Rosary — we are now on a first name basis — we are a family in the Blessed Mother's heart."

Even with the best of intentions, it is difficult to help each other if we are unaware of each other's problems. This difficulty is compounded if we don't understand our own problems. The Living Rosary solves this dilemma in giving to us the vehicle through which we can share our problems, discover more about ourselves and others and receive counsel and advice.

I'm still chuckling over an incident that recently happened to me in my efforts to promote the Living Rosary. I happened to be attending weekday Mass at a local parish and had the good fortune after Mass to meet Fr. John, a dynamic yet kindly Jesuit priest, who had been conducting a week-long retreat at the parish.

In the course of our conversation, I mentioned to him my work with the Living Rosary and he in turn told me of his own involvement with religious radio broadcasting.

It was when I mentioned the pen-pal group that he said, "I like that pen-pal group you've organized, Dr. Evers. The whole concept of people helping other people with their problems through prayer and sharing sounds great." Without waiting for any comment from me he continued, "Could you come over to the Parish School Library this Thursday? That's the day the retreat ends, and where I am planning to make a radio broadcast from there. I'd like to interview you, for the benefit of my radio audience, on the subject of the Living Rosary."

I really didn't feel comfortable thinking about the interview. Basically I get very nervous when I have to speak before an audience. As a child I used to stutter, and I'm always afraid the problem will return at an embarrassing moment. I knew the audience was a radio one, but the knowledge that it was a hidden one did nothing to quell my anxiety. I just hoped I wouldn't freeze.

The day of the interview finally arrived. Fr. John, sporting a cheery smile, met me in front of the school. I noticed a large white van parked some twenty feet from where we were standing. The call letters of a radio station were boldly written on the van's side panel. Feeling apprehensive, I remarked, "This looks like a pretty big operation, Father, and I don't mind telling you I get butterflies in my stomach just thinking about talking into a microphone."

"You do? That surprises me. You don't look like the type who would."

"Just goes to show how deceiving looks can be."

"Well, don't worry, Doc. This will be easier than you think. I'll warm you up with some questions which require brief answers. After you feel more at ease, feel free to elaborate on any point of the discussion you wish."

Surrendering to his encouraging words I nodded, and followed him through the school door into the library. The room, relatively small, was crowded with technical equipment. Three men and a woman were inside. Two of the men were arranging a battery of microphones on and around a rectangular table, and a third man was sitting at a small table in front of a huge, whirling machine. The woman was sitting before another machine with winking and blinking lights. Heavily insulated cables traced angulated patterns over the library floor. The whole scene looked very threatening.

Fr. John introduced me to the crew and explained that I was a little nervous, which generated comforting smiles, and directed me to one of the chairs at the end of the rectangular table. He then sat down, facing me, at the other end of the table.

The woman proceeded to pour water into two glasses, placing one to my right and the other to Father John's right. She then returned to her blinking machine.

"Dr. Evers," it was the woman who spoke, "would you please say a few words into the microphone; I want to check the audio."

As soon as she said, "say a few words," I felt my heart skip a few beats. "I hate this," I thought to myself. "Say? What does she want me to say! The first paragraph of the Gettysburg address — a prayer — a Bronx cheer..." Finally, after a few ponderous seconds of deliberation, I scratched on the microphone head, gritted my teeth as a cacophonous crescendo of noise reverberated throughout the library, and then very slowly and brilliantly said, "One — two — three — four."

"That's fine, Doctor, that's fine," I heard the woman saying. "The audio is picking you up very well." She repeated the same procedure for Fr. John.

The man responsible for the whirling tape machine spoke next. "Father, any time you're ready to start, we are."

Ready, who's ready? I thought to myself, as my throat muscles started to constrict.

Fr. John started talking. First he introduced himself, then me, then gave a brief description of the Living Rosary.

"And, Dr. Evers, please tell our radio audience, when did you first hear about the Living Rosary?"

This is it, this is it, I thought, the hour of decision. I wondered if anything more than a squeak would come out.

I hesitatingly answered, "The Spring of 1980." The thought went through my mind, "I did it, I did it." No stuttering, no stammering and no one was aware of my knocking knees.

Fr. John proceeded to ask more questions, each requiring a little longer response than the previous one. I noticed that my nervousness was disappearing and I was slowly calming down.

As the interview continued my answers became longer and longer. In fact, I was starting to enjoy it. Why, I even imagined my voice sounding like Gregory Peck, the famous actor. I continued talking, no — no — it wasn't Gregory Peck, why — I was convinced that I was sounding more and more like the late great orator, Bishop Fulton Sheen.

"That last remark you made, Dr. Evers, was most interesting and very well expressed indeed."

"You're right, Fr. John," I thought to myself, "it not only was well expressed, but rather excellently expressed."

By this time, I was really full of myself. I imagined I was in a miniature Cathedral and the audience of five plus thousands, enthralled by every sanctified word I uttered.

"And, Dr. Evers, tell our radio-audience, if you will, about this Living Rosary Pen-Pal Club that you have organized. It sounded so interesting to me when you first explained it."

Ah! The climax of my oration. My audience will be spellbound when I tell them about this. Clearing my now velvet-lined vocal cords ever so slightly and taking a small sip of water, I began. "Yes Father, it's all so very beautiful. What I do is send to each person a Rosary Calendar with the assigned decade they are to use. Also, I send them the names and addresses of the other members of their team." I found myself emphasizing the personal pronoun "I." I was most pleased with myself.

Fr. John interrupted me, "From what I understand, these people have specific difficulties. They may be elderly, lonely, and even ill."

"Yes, yes," I responded, "the elderly, the lonely and the ill are all linked through the U.S. Mail with each other, and then do you know what's one of the most beautiful things of all that I have them doing?" I put an extra punch on the word "I" this time.

"And what's that, Doctor Evers, please tell us, I know it must be something special."

I deliberately paused before answering and thought something like, "They could well canonize me for this" and then majestically said, "I have them praying for each other's intestines."

I could not believe what I had said. I meant to say, "for each other's intentions," but instead had blurted out a blooper and had all these good people praying for each other's intestinal tracts.

The technical crew in the converted library studio couldn't control themselves. They started cracking up with laughter. Fr. John joined them and threw up his hands, as my face changed several shades of red.

"Don't worry, Doctor, we can retape that portion."

"I hope so, I can't believe what," I started laughing at myself, "I just said."

"Think nothing about it. It happens all the time."

After several minutes had passed, and a sufficient amount of control had been regained by all, I started again and managed to get through the description of praying for each other's intentions. Fr. John then closed the interview with me and his radio audience.

"Well, that does it, Dr. Evers. I want to thank you for giving up you morning to come over here."

Still flustered and embarrassed over my blooper, and wishing I could crawl under the pavement to my car, I said a few parting remarks of thanks to Fr. John and the crew and left the building.

Just before getting into my automobile I picked up a brochure that had fallen on the ground. Looking at the cover I saw it was a schedule of Fr. John's retreat talks. Out of curiosity I looked to see what today's sermon was on. I blinked a few times to see if what I was reading was for real. The title, "We can all profit from our past mistakes," stood out in bold relief. "God is good," I thought to myself. It should have been entitled: "The humble shall be exalted and the exalted shall be humbled."

— 11 —

Rachel

"It must have been instantaneous." The telephone failed to mask the emotion in the emergency room physician's voice. "The police say she never saw the car, but just ran across the street without looking. She was chalk-white on arrival; there couldn't have been a drop of blood left in her poor little body. I'm sure the 'post' will show massive abdominal injuries, probably a ruptured spleen and torn liver."

As I listened to the physician, I could hear the screech of the brakes, the thud of the front fender, and could see her small, broken body lying on the bloodstained pavement.

I just couldn't believe it. Rachel was a beautiful, vivacious, eight-year old little girl. Her eye-catching dimples, bracketing an impish smile, could have melted the coldest heart. Now she was dead.

Glancing out of my office window, I recalled Rachel's routine visit a few days before. How free and graceful she looked skipping joyfully ahead of her mother down the graded sidewalk that exits our building. I detected the glint of parental pride and pleasure on the face of her mother, an attractive woman in her late thirties, as she attempted to keep pace with her fleet-footed daughter. And now the child was gone. I felt momentarily shattered and groped for words before replying, "I just don't know what to say — such a tragedy — such a terrible tragedy! Tell me, Doctor, is the family there?"

"Yes. The mother and her eldest daughter are here. The poor mother is hysterical. I gave her a sedative a short time ago and the daughter is trying to comfort her now."

"That must be Lisa; I'm so glad she is there. Those poor people. Thank you Doctor, for calling me. I'll go to their home this afternoon to offer whatever solace I can."

As I placed the receiver back on its hook, my mind drifted back to the death of our own daughters, Mary Ann and Kathy.

I recalled standing at our daughters' grave markers and promising myself that I would never abandon any parent in the hour of their greatest sorrow. No matter how uncomfortable it would make me feel, I would be there to share their grief.

Slowly, over the course of time our wounds healed, but to this day, two sensitive, loving scars remain.

I left the office earlier than usual because of my resolve to visit Rachel's mother. With a melancholy spirit, I drearily drove the four-mile distance to their home. How ironic; it had been such an ideal, sun-splashed June day, with cool Canadian air flooding the East Coast, yet it had been such a cruel and heartless day.

I stood for a few moments on the Cohens' front step, reaching for courage, and then gently knocked. Rachel's mother answered and without being asked, I stepped inside. Her ashen-gray face, laden with sorrow, met mine. Managing a weak smile she said softly, "Thank you for coming."

I whispered : "Mrs. Cohen, I am so terribly, terribly sorry."

She sat on a nearby sofa and stared emptily off into space. A tear-drop had formed on her cheek and like a guardian of the solemn moment, remained suspended.

"She never saw the car, Dr. Evers." Sobbing almost uncontrollably, she continued, "She — never saw it. Lisa told me — how happy she was — this morning."

"Mrs. Cohen, she could not have suffered. It was over in an instant."

I handed her a fresh tissue to replace the crumpled, saturated remnants she clutched in her hand.

Lisa quietly entered the room and sat on the floor near her mother's feet. We exchanged meaningful glances. The three of us, for a few endless moments, as in a holy sanctuary, sat motionless listening to and sharing the sacred silence.

I looked at them and said, "You know my faith is different from yours; I am a Catholic, and we believe in an eternal life with

God after death. In fact, we do not believe that happiness exists except after death."

Mrs. Cohen's face remained frozen in anguish as I spoke. "Oh! I wish I could believe that, Doctor. How I wish I could believe that."

At this point Lisa interrupted, "You know, Mom, something very peculiar happened this morning before the accident."

"What was that, dear?"

"Well, you know how Rachel always loved books and forever had one in her hand. Well, anyway, we were on our way to the library and had to pass a Christian book store. It's on one of the side streets. It has an open Bible in the window.

"When Rachel saw that big book in the window, Mom, you should have seen her. She first asked me what it was, and I told her it was a Bible. Then she asked me what it's all about, and I told her it was about God.

"You know what a good reader she was, Mom. Well, she must have spent fifteen to twenty minutes in the book store, turning the pages, reading and looking at the pictures. Every now and then as she read, a big smile would break out on her face. I kept motioning to her that we had to leave, and she would look up at me and mouth, 'Just a minute.' Finally, after I kept shouting at her to hurry up, she joined me.

"As we were walking to the library, I asked her what she had been smiling about. Had she read something funny in the Bible, or what? She suddenly stopped and looked at me with a question-mark expression.

"'No, Lisa, it wasn't funny. It just made me happy.'

"Then, Mom, you know how cute she was when she thought she had something important to say, how she would put her finger to her lips? Well, she did just that, and staring straight at me she said, 'Oh Lisa! I would like so much to go to Heaven and live with God forever. He must be so good!'"

Tears welling in our eyes, I grasped their hands and said, "Your Rachel is happier than you can ever realize. She lives forever with her God, our God. You must believe this."

No word was spoken. Mrs. Cohen just smiled wistfully as I slowly rose and, unescorted, silently left their home.

The next morning while in church attending daily Mass, I spotted in the pew directly in front of me a small book of religious verse. Opening the book, my eyes fell on the following lines:

> Our Creator dwelling in Mansions above,
> glances down on earth with looks of love,
> viewing a small child to call His own,
> He tenderly bends low to take her home.

— 12 —

Jimmy

Jimmy's tracheal tube was removed this morning. Both his mother and his father verify the almost impossible-to-believe fact that he said at least six words. "If anything, Doc," Mr. Murphy said, "he is saying more words now than I remember him saying before the accident."

Jimmy was in a mist tent because his voice was still quite hoarse, but whose voice wouldn't be after having had an endo-tracheal tube inserted in his windpipe for the past week. It seemed incredible, almost impossible, that little two-year-old Jimmy's small, frail body, now enveloped in a sea of mist, less than a week ago had been submerged for an estimated ten minutes in the family swimming pool.

I recall each syllable of the father's story of what happened. "Doc, I'll never forget that moment as long as I live. I was seated alone at the family dinner table, enjoying a T-bone steak. It was rare, just the way I like it. My back was to the swimming pool area and my wife was rounding up the children, who had eaten earlier, because a storm was approaching. It must have taken me a good ten minutes to savor and eat each morsel of that steak before I stood up, turned around and faced the swimming pool. I was looking through the sliding glass door at the approaching storm when I first spotted him. There he was, lying face down, floating motionless in the deep end of the pool, eight feet of water beneath him.

"The next four minutes are so confused and garbled I can hardly remember what happened when. I do know I frantically pulled him from the pool and threw him face down with enough force to bruise his forehead. I savagely started pushing in on his chest, trying by mere strength alone to force life back into him. He was blue, and limp as any ragdoll I have ever seen. I knew he wasn't breathing but, thank the Lord, I thought I detected a pulse. How I regretted not taking the cardio-pulmonary resuscitation course offered only months before. I was sobbing and screaming at the same time, 'Come on, Jimmy, breathe, please breathe.' Through my shouts I could hear the sound of a siren growing louder and louder. I learned later that my wife had called the rescue squad. The ambulance people told us afterwards that it took them only four minutes from the moment they received the call to get to our house. To me it was an eternity. Doc, you know the rest."

Indeed I do. It was just one week ago that I had received the emergency call. Gladys, one of the girls who operates our answering service, seemed unusually tense when she called me. "Dr. Evers, call Dr. Petro immediately. One of your patients just drowned." The urgency in her voice left me feeling numb and cold. I dialed the emergency room. It was 6:30 p.m.

The emergency room secretary quickly relayed my call to a central core area. A female voice answered. I knew it had to be Dr. Petro on the other end of the line; her obvious Slovac accent revealed her identity. She was an attractive woman who had been employed for the past few years in a full-time capacity as a pediatric emergency room physician. I had always been impressed by her competence and confidence. She spoke rapidly. "I have a little boy here, two years of age, with a history of being submerged in the family pool some ten to fifteen minutes. Doctor, he is breathing and that's about all. As he was being brought through the Emergency Room, he had a generalized convulsion which is now under control. I gave him intravenous valium and an anesthesiologist is entubating him now. He is going to need intensive care handling."

"I'll be there as soon as possible," I replied.

I recalled reading a superb article on brain resuscitation in drowning victims by a group of neurosurgeons in a recent pediatric journal who had a great deal of experience with this problem. I looked through my bedroom bookcase and thankfully located it. The article spelled out all the dangers in prolonged water immersion and precisely what course of action should be taken.

As I raced to the hospital, my mind paged through the article. Two organs received the brunt of the abuse, the brain and the lungs. Brain cells can be deprived of oxygen for no more than five minutes, then they start dying. This is a rather rapid process. In drowning, the brain receives a double insult: first, from the initial lack of oxygen and second, from the increased water ingested and inhaled. This is devastating to the brain, for now you have not only oxygen-deprived brain cells, but water-bloated brain cells.

Fortunately, however, in some drowning victims, the brain can survive much longer than five minutes, if the water is cold enough. Meanwhile, the lungs have their own battle to wage. Their main function is to deliver oxygen to the body and flush it of carbon dioxide waste. However water by this time has filled many of the terminal air sacs which accomplish this purpose, and the lungs have an overwhelming task on their hands with the functioning air sacs which remain.

To combat these problems, steps must be taken to aid the damaged lungs and brain. Using a respirator, as much oxygen as possible is forced into the few terminal air sacs and then into the body. To decrease the brain pressure due to swollen brain cells, the neurosurgeons suggest that the sick, swollen brain cells be placed at absolute rest. To do this the patient is given massive doses of barbituates, a medicine ordinarily used to induce sleep, to bring about a state of drug-induced coma; the body temperature is reduced to hypothermic levels by means of a cooling apparatus, and intra-arterial and intravenous tubes are inserted. Lastly, a small hole is made through the skull and a hollow screw, called a Richmond bolt, is inserted. The tubes — or lines, as medical jargon calls them — are used for delivering medications and for sampling blood chemistries. The Richmond bolt is used to monitor brain pressure. This was the ideal way to handle this problem.

Other disturbing thoughts whirled through my mind as I climbed the Beltway ramp into heavy traffic. The community hospital to which Jimmy had been hastily brought because of its proximity to the site of the accident is well equipped to handle most emergency cases; however, it did not as yet have an intensive children's care unit. The only hospital capable of intensive care was Metropolitan Children's, located twenty five miles away in the city.

Another problem that I faced was the lack of an experienced neurosurgeon who was capable of inserting a Richmond bolt and subsequently monitoring its care. Without an intensive care unit there was little opportunity for these otherwise excellent physicians to perform and monitor this procedure.

After snaking my way through a myriad of growling and coughing cars and trucks I reached the entrance to County General. I quickly parked the car and raced to the Emergency Room.

"Where is the little boy who was brought in here by ambulance, the one who drowned?" I asked the secretary at the entrance desk.

"Are you his doctor?"

"Yes," I impatiently answered.

"In emergency room one, Doctor."

I quickly found door number 1, the largest of the circularly arranged emergency rooms that surround a central core area. Directly inside, lying on an adult-sized examining table, was little Jimmy. He was motionless and in deep coma. I could hear, without the aid of a stethoscope, the gurgling water in his small lungs, as with irregular gasps they screamed for oxygen.

Preliminary life support measures already had been started. An intravenous tube inserted into Jimmy's right ankle vein was already operating, and an oxygen-delivering device was hooked up to the end of his endotracheal tube. Dr. Petro was bending over the boy's ankle, inspecting the intravenous site to make sure it was securely anchored to his foot and the pole with a bottle attached delivering life sustaining medications. Jimmy's parents, with lines of deep anxiety traced on their faces, stood frozen by their son's side. The situation was critical.

Breaking the silence, I said, "Let's transfer him upstairs as soon as possible, to the children's unit."

"I agree," Dr. Petro replied. "There is nothing more we can do for him here."

The next eight minutes were spent feverishly transferring Jimmy to the fifth-floor pediatric unit. After his arrival the entire unit became a hub of activity. Two nurses, an anesthesiologist, the excellent second-year pediatric resident, Dr. Wu, and I strategically placed ourselves about Jimmy's bedside. Adjustments were made in the endotracheal tube by the deft hands of Doctor

Brammer, the very capable, on-call anesthesiologist whose authoritative German accent, coupled with crisp commands, lent a sense of stability to the crisis.

Frothy, blood-tinged water and mucous welled out of the endotracheal tube. Jimmy's color by now was a mottled blue-gray and his condition was deteriorating rapidly.

"His lungs are like glue," Brammer snapped as he forced 100% oxygen through a manually operated ambubag. "Call the respiratory therapist and get the Born respirator immediately," he barked to one of the nurses.

My mind was spinning, for as the admitting physician I realized that the end responsibility was mine — and Jimmy was obviously dying.

Slowly and deliberately Dr. Wu suggested, "Dr. Evers, perhaps Jimmy should be transferred to Metropolitan Children's."

"Dr. Wu," I replied, "from the moment I first examined Jimmy in the Emergency Room I've been considering that option, but as ill as he is now he could well die in transit. I just don't think it's the right thing to do."

"Whatever you think best, Doctor."

"Do we have the capability to induce hypothermia or insert a Richmond bolt if I call a neurosurgeon?"

"No, we don't," replied Dr. Wu. "We don't have the monitoring expertise to attempt it, either."

"Well, we're just going to have to do the best with what we have, and furthermore..." my words were cut short by the floor nurse, who was signaling to me from the entrance to the unit.

"What is it, nurse?"

"Doctor, Jimmy's parents are very apprehensive and want to speak with you."

In my concern for the boy, I had forgotten the parents. As I approached them immediately outside the unit, their eyes met mine. "Mr. and Mrs. Murphy," I said, "Jimmy is critically ill and I am very concerned as to whether or not he will live."

"Dr. Evers," Mrs. Murphy replied, very carefully measuring her words, "I was very much present when Jimmy came into this world, and I want to be with him if he is going to leave us."

For the moment, I wasn't sure how to respond. Jimmy was ten feet away fighting for his life, and if his mother and father became hysterical it could well upset our objectivity and hence our treatment. I had seen Mrs. Murphy only a few times in the office in the past and also I had occasionally seen her at daily Mass. From these few encounters I had the impression she was a woman with much faith. In fact, they both were strong people. Looking at them I replied, "Mr. and Mrs. Murphy, follow me."

Mrs. Murphy immediately went to her son's bedside and, with great care not to interfere with those assisting Jimmy, she took his small, limp hand in hers and started softly chanting, "Jimmy you can do it. You can do it, little man. Your mommy and daddy are right here. You can do it." She continued to repeat this over and over.

"Doctor, look!" cried one of the nurses, "Jimmy has stopped breathing!"

For a few endless moments we all stood there paralyzed, refusing to believe that he was slipping away. I asked his mother to move back and then I frantically squeezed his chest in; I then relaxed, then squeezed again. I kept repeating this maneuver over and over, trying to force the fluid out of his lungs.

I said softly, "He's going."

His mother just as softly yet very deliberately answered, "No, Doctor, you're wrong. Jimmy is not dying. He is going to get well."

Out of the corner of my eye I caught a glimpse of the neonatologist who had just entered the unit to see what she could contribute. One of the few on hand with any great expertise in pulmonary physiology and pathology, she just stood by, shaking her head in despair. Jimmy's pulse had dropped from 100 to 60 beats per minute and I momentarily ceased my manual efforts. Then something wonderful happened. Jimmy, on his own, started to fight for life once again. His mother in the background continued her plea, "You can do it, little man, you can do it."

"Out of the way, everybody."

I spun around, wondering where the voice was coming from. Charging through the door was the respiratory therapist with the Born respirator.

"Over here, quickly" demanded Dr. Brammer. The machine was rolled to the front of the bed where, with grim determination and speed, Brammer hooked it up to the endotracheal tube. The machine took over, rhythmatically forcing 100% oxygen into Jimmy's lungs. The crisis had temporarily passed.

Looking at Dr. Wu I asked, "Have you started the IV mannitol and lasix?"

"Yes, they are running now."

Intravenous mannitol to shrink swollen brain cells, and intravenous lasix to facilitate removal of the excess water that had elsewhere accumulated in his body, I thought would help. All that could be done was being done, and though Jimmy remained in deep coma, with dilated pupils and absent reflexes, he seemed slightly improved. At least he was still alive.

Jimmy's father approached me. "What do you think his chances are, Dr. Evers?"

"That's a very difficult question to answer, Mr. Murphy, but for some reason I feel good about Jimmy. He's a fighter, you know, and your wife has great faith."

"Yes, I know what you mean." Mr. Murphy was stroking his hand through his son's hair as he spoke. "He is one tough little kid."

"We're doing all we are capable of doing, Mr. Murphy. The rest is really up to Jimmy."

"I know. I know you are. Thank you, Doctor."

It was well past midnight when I left the hospital. As I drove home I kept pondering over and over whether the correct decisions had been made. Now that Jimmy was stable, perhaps he should be transferred to Metropolitan Children's. After a few moments' reflection I discarded this thought. At 3:00 AM, how much better equipped would their unit be to handle Jimmy's problem? No, it was best to keep him where he was.

Enrico was on vacation with his family; I was handling the practice alone, and I knew about thirty-five patients would need my care the following day. Since it was summertime, a large percentage of the appointments would be for school physicals or camp examinations. There would be a few major problems — there always are — but Jimmy was my chief concern, and I hoped that the number of other problems would be minimal and easily solvable.

I didn't know how tired I was until I climbed into bed. When I am faced with medical challenges such as Jimmy's case I realize how heavily I rely on my partner. We function well as a team. We respect each other's wisdom and medical expertise, and I knew that if Enrico were here he would have some positive contribution to make. As I slowly drifted into sleep I felt a vague sense of uneasiness. I felt alone and isolated.

Much too quickly, 6:30 AM arrived The phone had not rung, so I knew that Jimmy was still alive. The early morning air was hot and humid. For the past two weeks the metropolitan area had been experiencing a torrid heat wave originating from the Gulf of Mexico. The weather, the traffic-ensnarled ride to the hospital, and my continued feeling of uneasiness all seemed to act as a harbinger of misfortune. I walked up the stairs to the pediatric ward and slowly opened the door to the continuous care unit. Hesitantly I entered. I was expecting the worst. The time was 7:15 AM.

Mrs. Murphy was seated in a chair beside Jimmy's bed, her back to me. When I walked to the bedside where Jimmy lay, I noticed immediately that his color looked improved over last evening. There was a tinge of pink in his cheeks, and he seemed to be in a deep sleep. I breathed a silent prayer of thanks.

"How do you think he is doing, Mrs. Murphy?"

"Oh, Dr. Evers, I didn't hear you come in. I must have dozed off."

Mrs. Murphy is an optimist, so I wasn't surprised when she said, "I think he is doing better doctor, in fact about an hour ago when I called his name I think he squeezed my hand."

"Really he did? That's great news. Will you excuse me while I check him over."

Jimmy's mother got up from the chair and moved aside. I sat in the same chair and spent the next fifteen minutes reviewing Jimmy's chart and giving him a physical exam. I was pleased with the recording of his vital signs. His blood pressure and his respiratory rate were normal. The physical exam was even more encouraging. His lungs were decidedly clearer than last night, although some distinct squeaks and squeals were still heard in both lung fields. When I squeezed the Achilles tendon of his right heel I had the distinct impression that his eyelids fluttered.

"Mrs. Murphy, it's too early to be absolutely certain, but I think Jimmy is definitely improving. Did you notice his eyes when I squeezed his heel?"

"Yes, I thought they moved, Doctor."

"I thought so, too."

If brain damage had occurred, the next twenty-four to forty-eight hours would tell how much. The fluttering eyes and the response to pain were favorable signs that Jimmy was waking up.

I told the mother that I had to return to my morning office appointments and unless I heard from the hospital about any problems concerning Jimmy, I would not return until this evening. As I retraced my steps down the hospital corridor to the elevator, I met Dr. Wu.

"Good morning Dr. Wu, good to see you. Did you get any sleep last night?"

"Good morning, Dr. Evers. No, I'm afraid I didn't get much sleep. We had three more admissions after Jimmy." Usually resident physicians look rather ragged after an all-night grind. Dr. Wu, on the other hand, looked cleanly shaved and freshly scrubbed.

"For someone who's been up most of the night you look pretty good. Have you had an opportunity to see Jimmy this morning?"

"Yes I did, about an hour ago. I think he is doing much better."

"Glad to hear you say that. I feel the same way."

The elevator had arrived and I was just about to step onto it when Dr. Wu asked, "Do you want me to reduce his barbituate dosage?"

I had forgotten that we had empirically started some Phenobarbital, a barbituate, last night on him after I left for home.

"Yes, yes Dr. Wu, I think you could safely do that. We may see a lot more favorable arousal response if we do. Call me if there are any problems."

With my partner out of town, the day was more hectic than normal, but I managed to wade through it. I had not heard from the hospital and I figured that was a good sign. In fact, I was even looking forward to my last appointment of the day — not because it would conclude my day at the office, but because it was a consultation with two parents that I was anxious to see.

The consultation was with the Cahills, a delightful couple and the loving parents of a three-year-old adoptive son, Seth. The Cahills were now seriously considering the adoption of a second child. I had been working with them all week, trying to help them in their decision. The adoption agency had called the Cahills two weeks ago to tell them that the agency had a two-month-old infant boy who could be placed in the Cahill's home. Unfortunately, however, the infant had a very stormy perinatal history. In addition to being four weeks premature, during his first two weeks of life the baby had developed a brain hemorrhage and meningitis. The fact that both of these complications occurred together carried ominous consequences.

The Cahills had told me in a previous conference one week ago that they really wanted this infant and they were perfectly willing to accept a child with physical handicaps. They were concerned, however, about their ability to care for an infant with severe mental incapacities. Mrs. Cahill's reasons were sensibly expressed, I thought, at the time of their last visit: "Dr. Evers, we just now don't know what the right decision is. We want to be fair to Seth, too, and a severely mentally handicapped child might be more than we can all handle."

Just before the Cahills' previous visit I had had an opportunity to talk at length with the neonatologist who had cared for the baby that the Cahills' were considering adopting. The neonatologist was able to give some encouraging news. The first bit of good news was that the brain hemorrhage was a minimal one, and a followup CAT scan of the brain, taken just prior to the baby's discharge from the hospital revealed that the hemorrhage had completely disappeared. The second encouraging piece of information was that the meningitis had been diagnosed early and that it had been treated vigorously.

This particular visit concluded with the Cahills saying that they would have to give the adoption some more thought and that they planned to call the foster mother who was now caring for the baby. I, in turn, promised that I would make every effort to obtain and review the baby's hospital chart.

Fortunately, I had received the chart three days before the Cahills' scheduled consultation. Unfortunately, in reviewing the chart I discovered that the infant had become badly jaundiced on the seventh day of life and the jaundiced level, as measured by a test called a blood bilirubin, had risen to a potentially high level. The condition was promptly treated with phototherapy, but still I worried that some of the bilirubin might have damaged the baby's brain cells.

The Cahills were already seated when I entered the consultation room. I could tell by their beaming faces that they had good news for me.

"It looks to me as if you have done some serious thinking and have made some decisions."

Mrs. Cahill laughed, "It's that obvious, isn't it. Well, we were able to contact the foster mother and she gave us some very encouraging news." Mr. Cahill was holding Mrs. Cahill's hand as she spoke.

"She told us she thought the baby was fine and that he is already smiling and holding up his head."

"Well, that does sound good, but how competent is this foster mother?"

Their smiles deepened, "She's been taking care of foster babies for five years, Dr. Evers. I would say that she is very competent. On the phone she sounded very level-headed, and we have just about decided on the adoption. Oh, by the way, did you get a chance to review the baby's chart?"

"Yes, I did."

"I can tell from your expression that you have some more information and it isn't good, is it?"

"You're right, I do have some information, and you're right again, it is a bit disturbing."

I then proceeded to explain in detail the high bilirubin level that the baby had developed and the possible neurological consequences. I told them also that the intense jaundice could cause hearing problems.

The conference ended on this discouraging note. I promised the Cahills that I would see if an auditory-evoked response test, which would give us valuable information about the baby's hearing, had been performed, and they in turn resolved to give further thought to the decision on the adoption of the baby.

As the Cahills were leaving the office they thanked me for taking the time to discuss the pros and cons of the possible adoption, and Mrs. Cahill turned to me, almost as if she were arguing with herself. "Dr. Evers, I feel that we could deal with a hearing problem, but I worry when you mention possible brain damage. But," she paused, and raising her eyebrows said, "still the baby is smiling, isn't he."

"Right, he is smiling and that's good. Let me see if any hearing test was performed. I will call you within the next few days."

It was about ten o'clock that evening when I finally made it back to County General. I had not heard from anyone all day long concerning Jimmy's condition. With confidence in the old adage that "No news is good news," I entered the unit.

Mrs. Murphy beamed when she saw me. "Guess what, Dr. Evers. Just an hour ago Jimmy opened his eyes and mouthed 'Mama.'"

"Are you sure?"

"Absolutely, Doctor."

"That's wonderful!" I replied.

I then approached the bed and proceeded with the same ritualistic examination. When I listened with the stethoscope, Jimmy's lungs, for the first time since admission, sounded perfectly clear. All traces of residual water had disappeared. When I squeezed his heel, as I did this morning, my heart jumped with delight. I saw the most beautiful sight in the world — Jimmy grimaced and then hissed through his endotracheal tube. I turned to Mrs. Murphy and told her what she already knew, that Jimmy's brain was functioning.

She was convinced that he was going to make a complete neurological recovery. I was not that optimistic, for I was still concerned that there could be some mental impairment, but I kept this thought to myself.

During the next twenty-four hours all my fears concerning Jimmy vanished. After the removal of his endotracheal tube his condition rapidly improved. In the ensuing weeks and months it was apparent that Jimmy had made a complete recovery without any neurological sequelae.

To make the next twenty-four hour period even more rewarding, the Cahills called to tell me that they had thought the adoption through once again and, regardless of the auditory response test results, they had definitely decided to adopt the baby.

Mrs. Cahill's last sentence before we hung up was, "It's that smile Dr. Evers, it's that wonderful smile that the foster mother says Gary has."

"Well," I thought, "if they have decided on a name, they must have decided on the child!"

The Cahills have since moved from the practice, but the last time I saw Gary he was about fifteen months old and was developing normally.

I like reflecting on the words of St. Margaret Mary, one of God's "little ones," to whom Our Blessed Lord revealed the riches of His Sacred Heart. She said, "Do not be afraid to abandon yourselves unreservedly to His loving Providence...rely entirely on God with perfect confidence in His goodness, which never forsakes those who, distrusting themselves, hope in Him."

Trust is everything. This is shown by the trust the Cahills and Mrs. Murphy had in God and the trust, because of this fact, that they would implant in their children.

How I love Pediatrics! Cases involving people like the Murphys and the Cahills, who live the words of St. Margaret Mary, make this specialty so wonderful and so rewarding.

With Stethoscope and Scapular

— 13 —

Sunburn

"Don't touch me, Dr. Evers; don't touch me!" Little four-year-old Faith Parks, her reddish hair smartly crowned with a single large silver barrette, was standing, clad only in shorts, on my examining table.

With a strained smile betraying her apprehension, she folded her arms over her chest in a vain attempt to hide her nakedness.

"You're not going to hurt me, are you, Dr. Evers?"

"Faith, Faith," pleaded her mother, "You know Dr. Evers is not going to hurt you, and you know I had to take your clothes off dear so he could see your rash." Turning to me she continued, "Oh dear, Doctor, I don't know why she acts like this."

"I don't think it's surprising, Mrs. Parks; some children are just more easily frightened than others. As for her modesty, it's only natural for little girls to act like this. Nature implants this gift very early in youngsters."

Not waiting for an answer, I approached Faith and said, "Don't worry darling, I'm not going to hurt you, I just want to look at your rash.

Starting to whimper, she begged me once again, "Don't touch me, Doctor, please don't touch me."

"I don't have to Faith, I'm just looking. Just try to relax." Moving a little closer to her, I exclaimed, "Why look, your rash is almost gone. You're almost well, isn't that good?"

"Yes! Yes!" Her eyes beamed as her fear, like a storm surrendering to blue skies, faded away.

"Can I get dressed now, Dr. Evers, can I get dressed now?" she pleaded. Faith still had her arms wrapped around herself, and I silently regretted not suggesting she put her undershirt on.

"Yes, by all means get dressed." Pausing, I continued. "And you know what?"

"What?"

"The best news of all, I won't have to see you again."

Jumping up and down with joy on the table, she went airborne and threw herself into the surprised arms of her mother.

"Oh dear, Faith, be careful. You almost knocked us over."

Faith, with a bustle of energy, insisted on dressing herself as with the aid of her mother she quickly put on her undershirt and blouse.

"Such enthusiasm," I remarked. "You've been so good, Faith, I wish I could give you something more than my customary kiss."

All I heard was "Could I..." The rest she whispered in her mother's ear.

"Well tell him, Faith; you can speak, you don't have to whisper." Then looking at me the mother said, "Oh dear, Dr. Evers, now she's playing Miss Bashful."

I thought to myself, kids do things like this, they are so natural, no phony boloneyness.

"Faith, what is it? You don't have to whisper in your mommy's ear. Just tell Dr. Evers."

"Well," she kept two fingers in her mouth while talking, but at least I could understand her. "Could I listen with your heart beater?"

"My what?" I shook my head in confusion, looking for an interpretation from her mother.

"She means your stethoscope, Doctor. She wants to listen to her own heart."

"Oh, sure," I laughed, "my heart beater. Of course, sorry Faith, I'm a little slow at times." Taking the ear prongs which were draped around my neck, I carefully inserted first the right then the left prong into Faith's ears, then I placed the bell of the instrument in her hand and directed it under her blouse to an area over her heart.

"Can you hear it going lubidy dubidy dub?"

She said nothing, but with an unforgettable look of discovery on her face kept shaking her head up and down. Then reaching for the ear prongs, she removed them and handed them back to me and said in a barely audible voice, "Thank you Doctor, I liked that."

"You're very welcome, sweetheart," and, kissing her on the head, I added, "God bless you darling. Good-bye."

"Bye, Doctor."

That afternoon an interesting incident occurred as if the morning were its prologue. I was working two examining rooms, shuttling back and forth between them, examining and prescribing for patients. The rooms' walls were of reasonable thickness and generally kept out most adjacent noise. Mrs. Scott had ten-year-old Matthew in, following a ten-day course of penicillin for infected tonsils.

A sweet, dear woman who had been bringing her covey of children to me since I first opened my doors, and who was usually gay and composed, this afternoon she seemed worried. Delicate lines laced her pale, thin face, reflecting her anxiety and with a wane smile she said, "Dr. Evers, Matthew doesn't look good to me. He's so pale and those dark lines under his eyes — ." She didn't finish her sentence, but just slowly and despairingly moved her head from side to side.

I had to admit that Matt, who ordinarily was a spindly, frail-looking lad anyway, looked a little bit worse than usual this afternoon.

"You're right, he does look a bit peaked, doesn't he? Hop up on the table, Matt."

Matt sluggishly obeyed. The exam immediately revealed the cause. His tonsils, large and boggy, were reinfected. For some reason, penicillin hadn't done the job.

It was about the time that I started listening to his heart that a raucous cough started blasting through the wall from the adjacent room. It startled all of us. "Cough, cough, cough." It was an Irish graveyard cough if I ever heard one.

"Oh dear," said Mrs. Scott, "and I thought my Matt was sick! She sounds perfectly awful."

I wondered how Mrs. Scott knew it was a girl; she probably was right. The cough had a certain female ring to it. Continuing to listen to Matt's heart, I thought I detected a noise I had never heard before. "Cough, cough, cough," it was difficult hearing and I couldn't decide if Matt had a problem or not. I had to do something about the patient in the next room.

"Mrs. Scott, excuse me for a moment. I'll be right back."

I quickly fetched one of the nurses and, explaining to her my difficulties, asked her to move the patient with the bad cough to a room at the far end of the hall. Returning to Matt and his mother, I proceeded with the exam.

"Cough, cough, cough." The sound was now muffled and distant, and looking at Matt I noticed a surprised expression on his face.

"What is it, Matt? You look puzzled."

"She sounds so much better, Dr. Evers, how did you fix her so quick?"

I laughed and answered, "Just gave her my magic medicine, Matt," and just as quickly added, "I'm kidding, Matt. All I did was move her to the end of the hall."

Smiling and putting my finger to my lips to indicate to Matt that he shouldn't ask me any more questions, I proceeded to complete my examination of his heart. Any new or strange noise would be reason for concern. One of the rare complications from inadequately treated tonsillitis is rheumatic fever with possible heart damage.

Taking my stethoscope, I slowly inched over his chest, listening first to the sounds of the heart valves opening and snapping shut, and then listening for any unusual noises between their opening and closing. I heard what I was listening for and breathed a sigh of relief. Despite the continuous coughing of the patient down the hall, it was quiet enough for me to be absolutely certain it was nothing more than an innocent heart murmur.

Turning to Mrs. Scott, I said, "His heart is fine, but the reason for Matt's sallow complexion and low grade temperature is that his tonsils are reinfected."

"But I gave him all the medicine."

"I'm sure you did, but sometimes even the most reliable of antibiotics let you down. Don't worry, I'll give him another one that should take care of it."

She seemed satisfied with my answer but then asked, "Why did you listen to his heart so long?"

I explained briefly about the danger of rheumatic heart disease, but assured her that the noise I heard was nothing more than an innocent heart murmur.

"Innocent? What does that mean, Doctor?"

"Well, it basically means he has a perfectly normal heart that makes a little swishing sound every time it beats, but it's absolutely nothing to worry about and he should be treated as a perfectly normal child."

"I'm relieved, very relieved, to hear that, Doctor."

"Cough, cough, cough." All during our conversation, the pulmonary lamentation continued.

"Dr. Evers, you've spent enough time with Matt and myself, you must take care of that poor girl."

I nodded in agreement, we exchanged good-byes, and with a promise from Mrs. Scott to call me in a few days with a report on Matt's condition, I departed.

Curious to see what the problem with the coughing girl was, I quickly strode the length of the hall and entered the examining room. In the center of the room stood a teenage girl, coughing almost uncontrollably. With each cough, her face became crimson blue in color and her whole body shook. She was petite in stature with long, blond hair and pretty blue eyes. She was clothed from head to foot in a long robe, much resembling a Hawaiian muumuu. For a moment she controlled her cough and smiled broadly in embarrassment over her inability to control her spasms.

"She's been doing this for the past two hours, Dr. Evers."

I immediately recognized her mother. She was a member of the church I attended, and on occasions, I had seen her at daily Mass. Her younger son had been in the office a few times in the past, but this was the first time I had seen her daughter.

"Oh, excuse me, Dr. Evers, this is my daughter, Teresa."

"Glad to meet you, Teresa, but sorry it's under such circumstances. That cough sounds terrible." Quiet for the moment, she nodded in assent.

"I'm going to have to listen to your lungs, Teresa, but I'm afraid I'm going to have to ask you to remove that lovely long gown you're wearing.

Staring at me with a look of surprise and dismay, she made no effort to follow my instruction. Her eyes darted from mine to her mother's and then back to mine again, silently pleading not to have to remove her outer garment. Her mother broke the awkwardness of the moment.

"Dr. Evers, you must forgive Teresa, you see she is embarrassed to remove her robe, because all she has on is her bikini bathing suit."

"Her bathing suit!" I replied in astonishment. We all grinned at each other at the absurdity of the situation.

"Were you swimming this morning, Teresa?"

"No, 'cough, cough,' no, I was just 'cough, cough' sun tanning at our, 'cough,' local pool."

"Why are you embarrassed?"

She continued to grin at me in a sheepish manner and mutely shrugged her shoulders, indicating she didn't understand, herself.

I shook my head in disbelief. "You feel naked in you bikini in a doctor's office, but you didn't feel naked an hour ago at the swimming pool?"

She didn't reply. Handing her an examining gown, I asked her to take off her robe and slip the gown over her bikini. I stepped out of the room while she did as I requested.

I waited a few minutes and then, knocking on the door, I inquired, "Are you ready, Teresa?"

"Yes," came a weak reply.

When I reentered the examining room, Teresa was sitting on the examining table waiting for me. The examination of her lungs revealed a small localized area of abnormal breath sounds, indicating a minimal pneumonia. In addition, the exam revealed a very skimpy purple and white striped bikini bathing suit.

"Well Teresa, the reason for your bad cough is that you have a patch of pneumonia in your left lung." Turning to her mother, I added, "An X-ray and blood count will be helpful to me in deciding treatment. I'll have the nurse take Teresa down to where both of these procedures can be done."

Within a few minutes the nurse was on hand with a wheelchair. Teresa, completely robed in the examining gown, awkwardly sat in the wheelchair. With both hands firmly grasping the chair's arms she was quickly whisked off by the nurse. Her mother remained with me in the examining room.

"Is her illness serious, Doctor?"

"No, no, not at all. It sounds much worse than it actually is. It's what's called 'walking pneumonia,' and with proper rest and treatment she should do well."

With a wry smile and upward flick of her eyebrows, Teresa's mother replied, "Swimming pool and sunbathing pneumonia sounds more like it."

"Yes, I know what you mean."

Her expression now sad, she replied, "I just don't know what to do. Teresa thinks I'm old fashioned about these things. And if I even mention something like immodest dress being a source of lustful thoughts and hence an occasion of sin for a young man..."

I interrupted and said, "And for older men, too."

"Yes, I know what you mean. Well, anyway, she just laughs and tells me that the times have changed." She sighed and added, "What's even worse is that her younger sister, Annie, has just started to swim and has been pestering me for a bikini-style bathing suit."

I replied, "Are you familiar with the Fatima apparitions?"

"Why yes I am, Doctor, although it has been some time since I have heard about them."

"Regretfully, you are right, they are rarely talked about nowadays, but nonetheless, they are more and more relevant than ever. At Fatima, the Blessed Mother warned people that immodest fashions would be introduced which would displease her Divine Son greatly. She told us to avoid such fashions, but the materialistic world has failed to listen."

The mother nodded her head in agreement as I continued. "Well, fortunately you and I know that Teresa's sense of modesty, although submerged, is still present. In a very peculiar way she demonstrated that to us this afternoon. You in a gentle, yet persevering, manner must guide her back to this virtue, holding the Blessed Mother up as a model. As for Annie, I would recommend that you just say no."

The mother's face brightened up as I spoke, and I almost visualized a cloud of confusion fading away.

The cough medicine I had instructed the nurse to give Teresa must have started to work, as now I heard only a few spasmodic coughs. The nurse opened the door to the examining room, and

Teresa rose from the chair, entered the room, and sat down. The nurse handed me the X-ray report and blood count results.

"Ah, just as I thought, your cough was sound and fury signifying nothing, if you will pardon the cliché."

Responding almost in unison, they inquired, "Why, what do you mean, Doctor?"

"Well, the blood count shows it's a viral pneumonia and the X-ray reveals a very small infiltrate. I think a little appropriate medication coupled with bed rest is all that is necessary, and in a few days you'll be one hundred percent better."

Smiles blossomed like spring flower beds at the favorable news. Looking at my watch, I realized I had spent more time than I had anticipated. With a few last minute instructions on diet and a follow-up exam, we said good-bye to each other. After closing the examination room, I paused to write a few notes on Teresa's medical chart. While doing so I could not help but overhear Teresa talking to her mother.

"Mom, what did you and Dr. Evers talk about while I was in X-ray?"

"I'll tell you all about it, dear, when we get home. I'll give you a hint, however. It concerns the danger of too much exposed skin."

— 14 —

April

I was in Examining Room Seven at the time, gently palpating three-year-old Mary's abdomen. Her mother, April, related to me that she had been up most of the night with intermittent tummy pains and a slight fever. It sounded like nothing serious, probably just a viral gastroenteritis.

Mary is an incredibly beautiful child, highly intelligent, and articulate for her age. Perhaps I exaggerate her attributes, but as her physician I feel strong emotional attachments to this little girl and her lovable young mother, April. In fact, April looked particularly pleasing to me eye this morning, for she exhibited all the signs of being pregnant with offspring Number Two.

The reasons for my very positive emotional attachment to this child and her mother are not difficult to understand. Three years ago a fateful series of events occurred involving me, April, then not married, and her parents.

As I recall, it was a beautiful spring morning with signs of new life exploding everywhere. Yellow daffodils dotted the emerging landscape and the perfumed smell of hyacinths hung in the air. It was a welcome relief from the unusually long, cold winter with its heavy snowfall and dreary gray skies that had engulfed the East Coast for the past several months.

Motoring to the office that morning, absorbing the sights and odors of spring, my mind drifted back to a telephone conversation I had had with April's mother, Mrs. Braxton, the previous evening. She was concerned over her teenage daughter who had been vomiting every morning or so for the past two weeks. She was sure it was infectious mononucleosis, which was reportedly rampant in her daughter's high school.

April was an unusually attractive, mature, young sixteen-year-old adolescent. Her manner was relaxed, her demeanor affable, and I had always enjoyed an excellent rapport with her. When it came to April's health, her unusually over-concerned and protective mother doted over her like a mother robin.

When I arrived at the office that morning, the nurse informed me that Mrs. Braxton and her daughter were already in an examining room. As I entered the room, April was sitting on the examining table, her legs dangling over the side with her elbows on her knees and her hands tucked under her chin. Two large saucer-like eyes surrounded with heavy eye shadow and a distinct eye-line met mine.

"Hi, Dr. Evers. How are you doing?"

Her face sparkled. She didn't in the remotest look ill to me. "What's the trouble, April? Your mother informs me you've been ill all week."

"Yeah, I've been vomiting every morning now for the past ten days, but I feel better as the day goes on."

Mrs. Braxton interrupted, "I'm sure it's infectious mono, Dr. Evers. Her school, as I told you last night, is absolutely loaded with it."

I thought to myself, infectious mononucleosis as a rule presents itself with symptoms of fever, sore throat, and fatigue, not with morning nausea and vomiting. However, April's symptoms can very definitely be the symptoms of an early pregnancy.

I was absolutely sure that her mother did not suspect this possibility. "Mrs. Braxton, you may be correct; it could be mononucleosis, perhaps complicated by a mild liver involvement causing the nausea and vomiting." A remote possibility, I thought to myself, as I attempted to buy a little time in deciding just what course of action and response I should take. I continued, "I would like to give April a thorough physical examination, and if you don't mind I think she would feel more comfortable if you left the room."

"Darling," Mrs. Braxton looked at her daughter, "do you mind if your mother leaves the room while the doctor examines you?"

"No, Mom, I'll be okay," she replied, half laughing as she spoke.

I slowly started my examination, leading up cautiously to the all-important question. I admit to being personally embarrassed by having to question adolescents about their sexual activities.

"How are things going with your school work, April?"

"Well, Doctor, I haven't been able to do much since I've been sick. Gosh, I feel lousy in the mornings. It's not until dinner that I even dare think of food. Do you think I could be pregnant?"

Thank you, April, thank you, I thought to myself, for making things easier on me.

"Do you have a steady boyfriend?"

"Yes."

"When do you think you may have become pregnant?"

"About eight weeks ago, Doctor."

"When was your last menstrual period?"

"Oh, I think about ten weeks ago."

Without responding, I proceeded with the physical exam. After finishing I looked at her and quietly said, "April, I think there is a good chance that you are pregnant."

I detected a trace of fear in her eyes as she replied, "Please don't tell my mother, Doctor."

Shaking my head from side to side I said, "April, that may be difficult. I don't think that decision is in your best interest, and I think you should at least discuss the matter with your mother. I know how anxious it must be for you, but..." She interrupted before I had an opportunity to finish. Almost despairingly, she blurted: "She will want me to have an abortion; I just know she will." I was shocked. This possibility had not even occurred to me.

"How do you feel about that, April?"

"I just don't know what to think. I feel as though there is life, I mean a baby, inside me, but I don't know what to do."

I was surprised by her answer. It showed insight and maturity. "April, I agree with you. There is life inside of you if, as I suspect, you are pregnant."

"How many weeks do you think I am?"

"I think about eight weeks. In fact, if you could see your baby at this precise moment, it would have a beating heart, a mouth, ears, and a nose, as well as arms and legs."

She looked distraught at my words, and my heart ached for her. "Doctor, I feel terrible. I have a girlfriend who goes to a female clinic and I think I could go there for help."

"April, provided it is a pro-life clinic, that sounds like a good idea. After you make your appointment you will be seen by a physician who specializes in Obstetrics. He'll take a complete history, give you an internal examination, and likewise will perform a pregnancy test. It's important that we confirm your pregnancy, although I am reasonably sure that you are.

"I understand fully why you feel as though you can't discuss the situation with your mother right now; I respect your decision and will not let her know my suspicions."

I prayed silently that Mrs. Braxton would not confront me with such questions as "Doctor, do you think she could be pregnant?" However, I didn't really believe April's mother had even considered this.

"April, after you get the results of the pregnancy test, do not make any decision on your own, but please promise that you will telephone me."

"I promise, I promise." I thought I detected a tear in her eye as she continued to nod her head up and down, repeating once again, "I promise, I promise."

I opened the examining room door and summoned April's mother. "Mrs. Braxton, I am not completely sure just what your daughter's problem is." This was a true statement since I was not one hundred percent positive of April's pregnancy. "It could be a vomiting flu bug, a strep bug, or then again it could be infectious mono. I've asked our lab technician to obtain a blood count and a mono test. I'll call you at the end of the day with the results."

The day passed without incident. I continued to mull over in my mind just what to tell Mrs. Braxton, as I was sure the blood count would be normal. I had an obligation, both to April not to betray her confidence, and also to her mother to offer her some reasonable explanation for her daughter's continuing loss of appetite and vomiting.

Our lab technician at that time was an attractive, competent, young lady named Doreen. Imagine my surprise when, finishing up with my last patient of the day, I heard Doreen's cheerful voice announcing, "Dr. Evers, guess what? April has a positive mono test."

I couldn't believe it. "Let me see the whole blood report, Doreen." Sure enough, her blood mono test was positive, but the rest of her blood picture lacked the typical elevation in white cells and abnormal number of atypical lymphocytes. Fortunately, she did have a few abnormal cells, and it was remotely possible that she had an extremely mild case of it coincidental with her probable pregnancy.

Knowing Mrs. Braxton would take the proverbial bait with hook, line, and sinker, I felt relieved as I dialed her telephone number. "Mrs. Braxton, this is Dr. Evers. I have April's blood results in my hand, and indeed, she does have a positive mono test with some atypical lymphocytes."

"That's just what I thought you'd say, Dr. Evers. I knew that mono test would be positive. Can I assume that she should stay home for the remainder of the week?"

Hoping that April's morning sickness would not last much longer, I replied, "I insist upon it, Mrs. Braxton; she needs rest and time to recover."

It was perhaps two weeks later that early one morning I received a frantic phone call from April's mother. "Dr. Evers," she stammered, "I don't know how to tell you this, but my daughter is two or three months pregnant."

"Are you sure, Mrs. Braxton?" I replied.

"Yes, absolutely. April went to a health clinic last week where a pregnancy test was performed which was positive. We must see you as soon as possible."

I feigned shock and surprise. Not knowing how much time I would need with April and her mother, or what course our conversation would take, I decided to cut my lunch hour and schedule them well before my afternoon hours.

On arrival at our office, Mrs. Braxton's cheeks were flushed and she looked slightly disheveled in appearance. Her hair was not immaculately groomed as was her custom, but wisps of it fell in haphazard array over her forehead. April seemed more composed.

I showed them into one of our large examining rooms. Looking me straight in the eye, and before I could utter a sound, April's mother announced, "Dr. Evers, you must understand one very important fact. Sixteen is much too young and immature to have a baby. I know April's father will agree with me. I insist that she have an abortion."

I did not immediately reply, but let her last words drift off into space. After some thirty seconds or so, I turned to her daughter and slowly asked, "April, how do you feel about what your mother is proposing?"

She replied sadly, "I don't know how I feel, Dr. Evers. I know I've disappointed my mother terribly and hurt her a lot. We still have to tell Dad. I feel so bad about the whole situation."

I asked, "Do you feel as though you have life inside of you?"

"I do, I do," she almost wailed in reply.

Turning to April's mother, I asked, "Are you Christian?"

"Dr. Evers," replied the mother, "indeed we are, and our church does not approve of abortions. They consider it taking a human life, but frankly, I don't care what our church says. This is a unique situation, and my daughter is very definitely not going to have this baby,."

Looking at them both I replied, "You know, April and Mrs. Braxton, I must make myself perfectly clear and let you know exactly how I feel and what my beliefs are. April is about twelve weeks pregnant. She has a separate, distinct life inside her at this moment. If you had X-ray and microscopic vision, you would see April's little infant almost perfectly formed with head, heart, hands and feet. In fact, the baby at this embryonic age has its own individual foot and hand prints. It is quite possible sucking its thumb right now. I honestly believe April's baby has as much right to life as any of the children I have seen in my office this afternoon."

They both were silent after my reply. I thought it a good moment to take a small pocket-sized *New Testament* that I had slipped into my examining gown pocket just before their appointment and offered it to them. I had made it my practice for a number of years to always keep some of them on hand, hidden away in my lower desk drawer for appropriate moments.

"Mrs. Braxton, April, I'd like you to promise to do one thing for me. Just accept this small *New Testament* of the Bible and set aside some time to be alone with the Lord. Let Jesus lead you through His words." Surprisingly, Mrs. Braxton offered no objection, and as they were leaving, she turned to me. The defiant attitude was gone. She smiled slightly and said, "You're a good man, Dr. Evers. We will pray over it."

About three weeks later, April called. "Dr. Evers, please may I fill you in on what's happened since I was in the office?"

"Of course," I replied.

"Oh, good! I want to tell you the whole story. After my last office visit, I returned home quite despondent, knowing I would have to tell my father that evening. Mom was a big help, and after dinner, finishing up with the dishes, we told him together. He was terribly upset, and if you only knew my father, you would understand. He was really devastated and kept shaking his head and repeating over and over, 'I just can't believe it. I just can't believe it.' After he calmed down, he simply insisted that the only logical thing, the only acceptable thing, was to have an abortion. He was so determined that I didn't dare suggest anything else."

"Because I was over twelve weeks pregnant, the only place legally I could have an abortion performed was out-of-state. So early last Friday, we left. The operation was scheduled for nine A.M., Saturday morning. We didn't say a word to each other the whole trip. I felt absolutely miserable. We checked into an inexpensive hotel near the clinic, and after a meal I can hardly remember, and television I cannot recall, we settled down for the night."

April took a deep breath as she continued her narrative. "Seven A.M. arrived much too quickly. Mom and I were on adjacent beds facing each other and my first words were, 'Mom, I just can't go through with it; I just can't kill my baby.'"

"I could tell by the expression on her face that she felt the same way. She replied, 'Let's get your father up, April, and get back home as soon as possible.'"

I breathed a silent prayer of thanksgiving as April finished her tale. "I'm so happy for you, April. Believe me, you have much to thank the Good Lord for, and I promise you, you will never regret your decision."

"I want to thank you, Dr. Evers, for all your help, and in particular, I want to thank you for that Bible. I've been reading it carefully and it was Jesus' words, 'Ask and you will receive, seek and you will find, knock and it will be opened to you' that made the difference. When I read that, I knew everything was going to be all right."

Abortion, the word makes me shutter. A strange paradox exists in our land. We are a people united in our battle against pain; we decry all forms of suffering, not only in humans, but in animals as well. We witness the unparalleled wrath by many vented against the helpless killing of seal pups. Both the pain and the bloody carnage that occur in the slaughter of these young animals revolts the human spirit. But some of these same people play the ostrich when it comes to the pain, the suffering, and the death of the intrauterine baby.

There is supportive evidence that the intrauterine infant probably experiences pain as early as the fifty-sixth day of life. Direct observation seems to indicate that fetal movements at the time are secondary to discomfort.

In first trimester abortions, a currette is used to scrape out the intrauterine baby, literally tearing him or her apart. In second trimester abortions saline is used. If the saline is accidentally injected into the mother's tissue, severe pain is experienced. How can anyone say that this same pain is not experienced by the intrauterine baby, regardless of which procedure is used?

April's tale happened almost four years ago. Now, looking at this beautiful child, I cringe inside. What if Mr. and Mrs. Braxton's death sentence had prevailed?

"April, dear mother," I said solemnly, "you have nothing to worry about. Mary just has a slight viral infection. The cramps will be gone by noon; she may have a little more discomfort, but she'll be fit as a fiddle tomorrow."

— 15 —

The Thirteenth Station

When time allowed, it was my habit to make the fourteen Stations of the Cross following Mass at the Cathedral. Its stations, massive in size and sculptured in pure marble, tracing the last events surrounding Christ's crucifixion and death, were both artistic and spiritual masterpieces. The finely chiseled expressions etched on each face begged for life.

It was the figure of the dead Christ in His Mother's arms that particularly held me spellbound. Standing before it in meditative silence, I could almost hear the tearless sobs of Mary as she cradled the innocent, blood-drained body of her dead Son in her arm. Upon leaving the Cathedral, with a kaleidoscope of fall leaves painting October trees and the joyous notes of school children's laughter overpowering my senses, I quickly forgot the morning meditation. The trip back to the office passed quickly, as I anticipated a light morning sprinkled with well physicals and a few ill children.

Mary Alice, our faithful receptionist, greeted me with the expectant news, "Doesn't look like too bad a morning, Dr. Evers."

"Good; I didn't get much sleep last night."

"Oh! What happened?"

"Would you believe it, Mary Alice, if I told you that our answering service called me at three AM to tell me of the birth of a healthy new baby?"

"They're not supposed to do that, are they?"

"No, they are not! It must be a new girl working for them. I'll call them later on today and see if I can straighten them out."

Mary Alice, not only our receptionist of many years, but my wife's dearest friend, was a remarkable woman.

Her dark brown eyes and raven black hair hinted of her Italian ancestry. Jean used to lament, "If only I could get a tan like Mary Alice."

She possessed boundless energy and unlimited industry. If she wasn't answering the phone or signing patients in or out, she was filing charts. For a person so thin, you wondered where she stored it all.

But most of all, it was her magnetic personality blessed with an infectious smile that marked her apart from others. She didn't realize it, but her smile was her ministry in life and her gift to others. Even after she was taken away from us, we who loved her would always remember her smile.

I was not involved with the first patient more than five minutes when Mary Alice interrupted me over the office intercom.

"Dr. Evers, Mrs. Gleason's calling you from County General's Emergency room. She seems terribly upset."

Mrs. Gleason, an attractive young mother, gracious and gentle, had been in the office a few days ago with her tow-headed little boy, Dickie, for his annual physical. Smiling to myself, I recalled in particular the pride in this mother's eyes retelling little Dickie's latest four-year old feat. I shared her admiration. He was a bubbly, bouncy little tyke who, with the agility of an Alpine mountaineer, would leap up on my examining table before he was even asked.

Most four-year-olds viewed certain parts of the physical exam with apprehension, but not Dickie. It was just a joyous game to him, and I did my best to oblige. Probing his stomach, I would inquire, "Let's see if I can find out what you had for breakfast this morning." A laugh would erupt from Dickie as he waved his head from side to side mutely implying, "I dare you, I dare you."

Then I would glance at his mother for help and she would mouth the morning menu.

"I think I feel some scrambled eggs here. Yes, I'm sure I do." Ripples of laughter from Dickie would ensue. Proceeding to a different area of his abdomen, the litany of discovery continued.

"Oh! What do we have here? Toast with some jam." Dickie's eyebrows arched cutely upward and with a pixie grin he giggled once again and said, "What kind of jam?"

His mother had already clued me in, but I feigned ignorance. "Let's see; I think it must be strawberry jam."

"No, no, not strawberry," Dickie laughingly replied in a falsetto voice.

"Raspberry?"

"No! No!" a staccato laugh punctuated each no.

"I know what it is, it's peach jam. Yes, I'm sure it's you mom's homemade peach jam."

"Yes! Yes!" He howled with glee at the discovery.

The rest of the physical exam proceeded without incident, and when I announced to them both that he was in perfect health he jumped off the table, wrapped his arms around my legs, and said, "I love you, Dr. Evers."

That was less than three days ago, and now his mother was calling me from our local hospital's emergency room. Mary Alice said it sounded urgent. With an ill feeling, I lifted the receiver to my ear. "Mrs. Gleason, this is Dr. Evers. What's wrong?"

"Dr. Evers." She was sobbing, "Dr. Evers — the doctors here — tell me — Dickie is — is — dead."

I was momentarily stunned and groped for a meaningful reply.

"Dead, are you sure they said Dickie's dead?"

"Yes...yes."

"Can you tell me what happened?"

"I just — just got — here Dr. — Evers"; her sobs were heartbreaking.

"They say he — was run over — by — a tractor lawnmower — at school this — morning."

My mind chilled at the thought of massive rotors cutting his poor little body into fleshless ribbons.

Mrs. Gleason's sobs died to barely audible sights. "Doctor, I know you must be busy, but could you possibly come here? I just can't bear to look at his body — and — I want to be sure it's him."

"Yes, yes, certainly Mrs. Gleason, I will leave at once."

Not cognizant of the time, I immediately left the office and quickly motored to County General Hospital.

Parking my car in the Emergency Room's adjacent parking lot, I walked swiftly toward the entrance. A voice within me — a voice I knew I could not trust kept repeating, "Maybe it isn't Dickie; maybe it isn't Dickie."

With an anguished heart, I opened the door and entered. Not wanting to know, I approached the receptionist to ask where the mother of the young boy who was tragically killed this morning might be. Sadly and silently she pointed to a glass-enclosed waiting room. Looking in the direction to which she was pointing, I immediately saw Mrs. Gleason sitting on a chair despondently staring at a small flowering plant. As I approached her, she saw me and rushed toward me crying. "Dr. Evers, Dr. Evers, it was so good of you to come."

Instinctively I placed my arms around her, and with her head momentarily buried in my shoulder I gently comforted her. Looking at her tear-stained face I softly said, "I'm so terribly, terribly sorry, Mrs. Gleason."

Hardly hoping, almost completely despairing, she replied, "Make sure it's him; make sure it's Dickie."

An emergency room nurse had been standing just out of sight waiting for me. Without speaking, she beckoned me to follow her. Catching up with her I inquired, "Can you tell me what happened?"

"From what I understand, about three hours ago at his nursery school, the maintenance man was mowing the grass with one of those huge tractor lawnmowers. The little boy broke away from a group of young children that the teacher was guiding to the playground and ran directly in front of it."

"How terrible! Why couldn't the teacher stop him?"

"It happened so fast. Apparently, he spotted a little puppy dog in the grass just on the other side of the lawnmower; it was over before anyone realized what was happening."

I groaned silently to myself as we approached a narrow green metallic door.

"He's right inside this room."

The nurse briefly hesitated, then opened the door into a small darkened room.

The nurse switched on the lights, and I saw that a large stretcher with wheels completely dominated the room. On top of the stretcher lay a small sheet-draped body. The nurse drew back the sheet.

It was Dickie; there was no doubt about it. His hair was thickly matted with blood and closer inspection revealed a cruel gash extending half way around his head. Even his body had not escaped the merciless blades, for a deep penetrating wound had pierced his right chest. I felt momentarily shattered and fought back tears. He looked so innocent, so alone, and so blood-drained. The nurse reverently covered his little body, and with heavy steps I returned to the waiting room.

His mother was waiting for me and asked, "It's Dickie, isn't it?" I sadly nodded my head yes. She started sobbing deep, hopeless sobs.

Holding her head and gazing at her, for a brief moment I could hear through the tunnel of time, the echo of nails and the thud of a lance, and could see reflected in her tearless eyes the aching, sorrowful heart of another mother on Calvary's hill — a mother who, like Mrs. Gleason, had no more tears remaining to shed for her dear little boy. Somehow I felt peaceful inside, because Calvary's Mother would soothe the pain of this mother and Mrs. Gleason would find the strength and courage to go on because of the example of Jesus' own Mother who is, and never ceases to be, our mother, too.

With Stethoscope and Scapular

— 16 —

Lori

Four-year-old Lori should hold symposiums for foreign ambassadors. Her effervescence and sociability are boundless. Today was no exception. In the office with her two brothers she was politely making rounds, trotting up and down the hall shaking hands with Esther, our lab technician, Ann and Mary Ann, our Tuesday nurses, and finally me.

"Hello Doctor." she offered her tiny hand to me as I stooped over and gently accepted it.

"Hello Lori, are you sick today or just visiting?" I asked.

"No, no sick," she replied.

"I see, just visiting. Good, I'm glad."

Her father, standing in the doorway of the examination room, holding the youngest one, Anthony, in his arms, smiled broadly.

"She's always like this Dr. Evers, even with perfect strangers; she runs up to them with happiness written all over her face and holds her hand out."

I nodded and, sweeping Lori up in my arms, gave her a loud kiss on her right cheek. Throwing her arms around my neck, she giggled with joy. Giving her an affectionate squeeze, I placed her back on her feet, from which point she continued her merry romp.

"She loves everybody, doesn't she, Mr. Santelli?"

"Yes, and sometimes it worries me."

I knew what he was referring to. Little Lori trusts absolutely everybody. She doesn't know the meaning of the words fear and danger, and furthermore, she couldn't comprehend anybody actually wanting to harm her. But so many children with Down's Syndrome are like that. They are filled with perfect, trusting love toward everybody.

Down's Syndrome was unmistakable from the day of her birth; the slightly flat nose and slightly slanting eyes, the short thicker fingers, the tongue larger than normal and the loose skin fold at the nape of the neck. There just was no doubt about it. Yet now, her captivating personality all but hides these physical defects.

I vividly recall the difficult time I experienced when Lori was born, explaining to Lori's mom and dad the future mental and possible physical limitations she faced. Some children are more severely afflicted than others, and I always like to be as hopeful as possible without painting a picture of false expectations. That was three years ago, and since that time her parents and I have grappled with her three narrow encounters with death and a major heart operation. Little Lori has had to walk a dark and dangerous path in her short life, but in reviewing her past year of relative good health, she appears at last to be breaking into sunlight. However, I should let Lori's father tell the story, which he wrote down a short time ago. He gave me a copy that I have carefully filed away. Already I have been able to beneficially use it for another family who has a child with Down's Syndrome. It is a tale of courage, determination, and faith.

God's Gift of Love

"My wife and I were very happy as we prepared to go to the hospital. Our second child, although four weeks early, was soon to be born. Sixteen hours later the baby had not come. The prolonged labor was starting to take its toll on Gay. Her doctor, moreover, had become quite concerned at that point because the baby appeared to be in serious danger. He decided to perform a caesarean section. I was worried, and yet relieved. I remember thinking that my wife's difficult pregnancy finally would be ending.

"Two hours later her doctor came to me with the news. Gay was fine; the baby was a girl; her heart had stopped beating momentarily during delivery, but she was okay now. Then he told me: 'Your little girl has Down's Syndrome.' I really knew little about this genetic affliction. The doctor told me our baby would be mentally retarded. She would also suffer from a number of physical ailments. She might have hearing, eye, and respiratory problems. Her poor muscle tone would also cause her difficulties. This was only the beginning, as we later fond out. The baby's immune system was deficient in warding off diseases. Finally, she had a serious heart defect. I was stunned. I asked myself: 'How could God do this to us? What had we done to deserve this? How could He allow an innocent child to suffer and go though life with such infirmities?' I felt abandoned, and a terrible depression settled over me.

"Gay's doctor, however, was compassionate and attempted to give us encouragement. Although we were told later by others that we could give the baby up, we never considered this to be an option. Lori was our daughter. I had decided to care for her, but could I love her as I did my son, who had seemed so perfect from the moment of his birth? The answer, I thought, was no. In fact, I was initially reluctant to get close to her and even felt it would be better for her to die.

"Although she was in stable condition, we decided to baptize her while in the hospital. I was allowed to bring our one-year-old son to witness the administration of the Sacrament by our parish priest. Stevie, upon seeing his new sister with his mother, toddled as quickly as he could to their bedside and exclaimed with wild excitement the new word he had learned, 'Baby!' He was overjoyed. I later felt ashamed of myself, for he immediately had loved and accepted this new child. Could I do anything less?

"We took Lori home eight days after she was born. Gay and I prayed for God's help. We were still overwhelmed by what we considered a tragedy. Our attitude was soon to change. Four weeks after Lori's birth, I found myself speeding through traffic to the hospital with Gay next to me, cradling Lori in her arms. The baby, from all appearances, seemed to be dying. Her breathing was labored, she was listless, and her color had turned an alarming gray. I prayed all the way, begging God not to let her die. How ironic, for less than a month before I had almost wished for her death. For days Lori hovered between life and death. She had mysteriously come down with a severe case of salmonella and was having frequent episodes of bloody diarrhea. Gay and I were distraught, yet I had a strong conviction that she would not die. God, I thought, had given Lori to us for a reason, and He was not going to take her from us now. The disease was devastating, and the doctors in the first few days were not all that encouraging about her chances for survival. We asked our relatives, friends, and parish to pray for her. God answered these prayers. She came home after nearly four weeks in the hospital, a tiny five-pound baby with marks and scars over her body from the life support system that had sustained her.

"Gay and I knew God had given us a miracle in preserving Lori's life. We also knew He had brought us closer to her. This was a gift, for a bond of love now existed between us and our little daughter. This bond grew stronger during the following months. Thoughts of rejection had evaporated into acceptance and overwhelming love.

"Lori's suffering, however, had not ended. More serious medical problems arose. Gay and I spent countless sleepless nights trying to care for her the best we could. We also experienced the pain and anguish of seeing her come perilously close to death again and again. More hospitalizations came, including one for delicate open heart surgery. In her first 21 months of life, Lori had been seen by 90 different physicians. All the while Gay and I sought God's help. We really had no choice, for He was our only refuge. Repeatedly we asked Him to spare her life, to guide us in knowing how best to care for her, and to grant us His grace and strength to sustain us. We also turned to Mary and the Saints and asked for their intercession. Our prayers have always been answered, but not necessarily in the ways we wanted. God in His mercy has granted us many miracles, for Lori has survived all the illnesses she has encountered, even though the odds were against her.

"Lori is now two and a half and a vital and inseparable part of our family. I cannot envision the family without her. Once I thought of her as a possible burden, now I see her as a wonderful blessing. The pure love I see which Lori gives to our family and to others who know her, and which is returned to her, has become for me a great source of happiness. This love far outweighs any pain and sorrow that I have had as a result of her problems.

"Gay became pregnant once more shortly after Lori was a year old. Our doctor told us that we stood a good chance of having another child with Down's Syndrome. Admittedly, we were anxious, but we resolved to place our trust in God. Because of the love we had for Lori, we decided that should we have another child with Down's Syndrome, we would love, accept and care for the baby as we would any other child of ours. Lori had taught us that lesson. In June of the following year God blessed us with a healthy boy.

"The crises we have faced have brought Gay and me closer to each other and closer to God. Caring for Lori has taught me what true love is all about and how dependent we all are upon God and each other to sustain us through life's difficulties. I have often thought that she was sent to us, in part, to strengthen my faith and to assist me on the road to salvation. Beyond this, God has another purpose in mind for Lori. Already she has touched the lives of so many. This courageous, happy, and now vibrant little girl has shown us and those that have come in contact with her that being handicapped is not a tragedy. She is a special child, a special gift from God with such a special love that makes it a joy and a privilege to be her father."

I have read Mr. Santelli's story many times, and each time it thrills me to realize that by being Lori's physician I have been a small part of it. Lori's parents are remarkable people. They have great trust in the goodness and the preciousness of life. I recall when Mrs. Santelli was pregnant with their youngest, Anthony, and she reported to me her reply to the doctors who advised that she have an amniocentesis. "Why do it at all," she said, "it will make no difference what you find out, we'll accept whatever God has prepared for us."

Now Anthony's Dad was holding him in his arms while we continued to enjoy Lori's frolic up and down the hall.

"Come on, Lori, settle down," said her dad, "the doctor has to examine Anthony."

While Mr. Santelli moved inside the examination room, one of the nurses corralled Lori and brought her into the same room. She quickly quieted down and stood beside her dad, who was sitting down in a chair with Anthony in his lap.

Anthony had had a nasty cold a month or so ago and developed an ear infection of the right ear. The infection cleared up nicely with antibiotics, but at the time of his last visit I noticed that fluid had accumulated behind his right ear drum. This is not an uncommon complication and usually clears within three to four weeks. Rarely, fluid will not clear and a thick, gummy substance remains behind. If undetected, a hearing problem could result. He was in the office today for re-examination.

"Good to see you, Anthony, are you going to let me see your ear?"

Anthony, at the mere sight of my otoscope, started crying. The doctor's office is not his favorite place. Today his reaction to the otoscope was neither unexpected nor surprising. He started crying pitifully. I sat on a chair directly opposite him and his dad and very carefully started to insert my speculum inside his right ear. He immediately and predictably started thrashing his head from side to side trying to fight me off.

"Anthony," said his father, "don't move so much. How can you expect the doctor to see if you're getting better?"

I spied Lori out of the corner of my eye during the developing scenario. Like a perfect little mother she was holding one of Anthony's hands and gently patting it, trying to comfort him. Like magic, her action seemed to have a calming effect on her little brother and he settled down just long enough to enable me to see what I was after.

Taking the speculum out and looking at Lori I said, "Lori, thank you, thank you very much. I was able to see your brother's ear and the fluid is almost 100% gone."

"Oh," said the father, "I'm glad to hear that. Will he have to be seen again?"

"No, he's cured."

"That's good news, Doctor." Then looking at his daughter he continued speaking. "Do you know, Doctor, Lori's a big help to her mother and father around the house. She is very, very sensitive to both her brothers' needs and when she hears them crying immediately rushes to them and tries to comfort them."

I replied, "Lori, Anthony's awful lucky to have you as a big sister."

Lori twisted bashfully on her heel and smiled broadly.

"And you know what else she does, Dr. Evers?"

"No, tell me."

"She knows how to make the Sign of the Cross and blesses her brothers each night before they go to bed."

Lori heard the word "cross" and started to bless herself, and then pointing at me said loudly, "Doctor, Doctor."

Her dad laughed, "She wants you to bless yourself."

I did as she asked and replied, "Lori, you are such a good girl. How Jesus must love you."

Lori seemed to understand the importance of the word "Jesus," and smiled once again.

"And one more thing I must tell you, Doctor."

"What's that?"

"She has a very forgiving heart and she shares beautifully. If her brothers push her or grab something away from her, she lets them know in her own way that they are forgiven. Of course, this does not happen before their mother or I correct the boys. And she is always sharing her toys with them."

"She is a wonderful child, Mr. Santelli."

"I mean this sincerely, Dr. Evers, every family needs a child like Lori."

The visit was finished and Anthony, detecting that I was no longer a threat, started jabbering happily in anticipation of his leaving. I was just about to say good-bye when Mr. Santelli inquired, "Dr. Evers, Gay and I are aware of your involvement in Natural Family Planning; do you know where we could get some information on it?"

"Certainly, I have some information in my office library."

"I'm pleased to hear that. You know my wife and I want to have another child and," he stopped in reflective silence for a moment and then continued, "and this may sound strange, but at times we almost wish for another child like Lori."

Having been given the privilege over the past three years to have a peak into the hearts of these wonderful parents, his request and the reason for it didn't sound strange at all.

"Mr. Santelli, what you're saying sounds not only logical, but beautiful, to me. Wait a minute and I'll get you the information you're after."

One of the great benefits behind NFP is that with the added knowledge given a married couple in respect to the wife's fertility, they know the best time to engage in marital love if they want to have a child.

Handing him some information pamphlets that I had obtained from the Couple to Couple League, an organization located in Cincinnati, Ohio that promotes NFP, I said, "You know the bible said it all years ago, 'There is a season for everything...a time for embracing, a time to refrain from embracing.'"

Mr. Santelli smiled, accepted the literature, and said, "Well, we are very interested in the former part of that biblical quote and would like to add one more word, fruitful embracing."

Smiling in return, I replied, "Amen to that, amen to that."

In due time Mr. and Mrs. Santelli had their fourth child, a beautiful little girl who they named Elizabeth.

I recall one occasion when little Elizabeth, sporting a gorgeous smile, was in for her four-month-old physical exam. Mrs. Santelli had tied a pink bow in her hair and she, unlike her brothers and her sister at the same age, was a perfect doll throughout the examination.

"She gets an A-plus on her physical examination, Mrs. Santelli. She is a perfectly normal four-month-old little girl. Her developmental milestones are, if anything, ahead of normal."

"Thank you, Dr. Evers. All the children love her, and her daddy and I feel so blessed."

"Mrs. Santelli, you and your husband have such a profound, yet simple, trust in God; little Elizabeth's arrival and good health do not surprise me at all. However, there is one thing I think I am going to do."

"Oh! What's that, Dr. Evers?"

"Well, when you bring her in for her six-month-old physical exam, I'm going to erect bleacher seats in the examination room and provide cotton candy."

Mrs. Santelli laughed and asked, "Oh, why are you going to do that?"

"Well, I intend to invite her two older brothers and sister, and while they sit and enjoy their cotton candy they can see how a young patient should behave during a physical examination."

Elizabeth's mother, not to be outdone in one-liners, replied, "We'll be there. I just hope the tickets aren't too expensive."

— 17 —

The Widow's Mite

He glanced up and saw the rich putting their offerings into the treasury, and also a poor widow putting in two copper coins. At that He said: "I assure you, this poor widow has put in more than all the rest. They make contributions out of their surplus, but she from her want has given what she could not afford — every penny she had to live on."

There was a message on my telephone call box from Bill Altman, an attorney friend of mine who has been helping me with the CPR Corporation. The initials, CPR, stand for Colbert Poor Relief, a corporation I formed to help the poor. It is named in honor of my grandmother, who had been so instrumental in my own personal devotion to the Rosary.

Forming the corporation evolved from my work with the Living Rosary. The many missionaries, particularly in Africa and India, to whom I had sent the information on the Living Rosary, responded that they thought this prayer form was very useful among their parishioners and new converts. But also they told me about their hunger and their need.

I had already sent information on the Living Rosary to thousands of people in the United States and hundreds of people in Canada. They, in turn, had told me how helpful it was, not only in temporal favors received, but also in uniting their parishes and families in prayer.

I truly believed the Blessed Mother wanted the Living Rosary members in the affluent Americas to help their less fortunate brother and sister Living Rosary members in Africa and India.

In fact, about two weeks ago, I had sent out my first solicitation letters to about two hundred members to ask for their help.

I was sure the reason Bill was calling me was to give me some news on the tax-exempt status that I was trying to obtain for the corporation. His assistance had been invaluable so far, and I felt if anyone could help me with this final phase, Bill would. Dialing his number, I held the phone to my ear. It rang several times before a recorded voice answered, saying that all lines were busy. While continuing to hold the phone, I surveyed the top of my desk and noticed that my morning mail had arrived. Happily, I noticed several responses from my first solicitation letter that I had sent out on behalf of the CPR Corporation.

While the telephone serenaded me, I scanned a copy of the solicitation letter that I had sent out.

The highlights of the letter read as follows:

> Dear Living Rosary Member,
>
> I am writing to you because of your interest in the Living Rosary. Many of those to whom I sent the information on the Living Rosary were Missionaries and Religious working in distant mission posts. They have enthusiastically adopted this prayer and find it very useful, but in their letters they also tell me of their hunger and their need. I would like to share with you some of their responses.
>
> Father Beyene Hailu in Ethiopia told me, "We have a very hard time here with the victims of famine and hunger. Most of the day I had to attend the funeral ceremonies in the parish. As you might know from the mass media, people are just dying because of famine. We see many tragedies and heart-touching happenings every day. Deaths are common and we are just frustrated burying bodies. At times one family all together. Do you know of any association which can help the victims of famine around the world? It would be really God's blessing for the dying if you can make a request on our behalf.
>
> "Be it big or small, any donation is useful for the poor here. Checks reach us quite easily in an ordinary mail. Sorry for bothering you too much, but I have nowhere to turn to and I can't see any good keeping my mouth shut while seeing Christians die."

Father Gregory Koottummel, a parish priest in South India told me, "The number of groups of the Living Rosary are on the increase. It is spread in various wards of this village. An active member of the Living Rosary has joined a religious congregation. Moreover, she was one of our Sunday School teacher. She joined the Daughters of the Heart of Mary.

"Now we are experiencing heavy rains. The poor around this area are starving having no work.

"Remember a member of the Living Rosary who is bedridden. He is very old."

Father Karikampally, from Nilgirls, South India says, "Greetings, this is a remote village. People are poor and they could be destroyed by wild elephants, boars, etc. Please do recommend me and my poor children especially to some of your good, generous friends. They are always asking for school fees, books, uniforms, clothes, etc."

These missionary letters would touch anyone's heart, I thought to myself. If any group of people in the whole world was living out the mystery of redemptive suffering, it was these poor missionaries and the parishioners they serve.

The closing paragraphs of the solicitation letter, I believe, capsulated the whole idea behind charity to the poor. They read:

The function and purpose of the CPR Corporation will be to live out the words of Our Lord Jesus when He will say to us someday: "For I was hungry and you gave Me to eat; I was thirsty and you gave Me to drink; I was a stranger and you took Me in; naked and you covered Me."

Just as CPR is used in medical emergencies to preserve heart and lung function, I hope and pray that the CPR Corporation can do its part in diminishing the heartache of hunger and the suffocation of poverty among these poor people. Let your heart decide on how you can give.

I was musing over this last paragraph and still listening to the recorded music when suddenly it stopped and Bill came on the line. "Joe, sorry to keep you waiting so long, but I was tied up with a long distance call that I couldn't interrupt." Before allowing me to respond, he continued,

"Got great news for you, Joe. I talked to an Internal Revenue man yesterday who said all the papers were in order and your tax-exempt status should be coming through the mail in a few days."

"That's fabulous, Bill. I really don't know how to thank you for all you have done."

"Don't be silly, Joe. It's my pleasure and don't forget to keep me informed on your response to your first mail out."

I was very excited over the news of the tax-exempt status and now knew that the CPR Corporation was at long last off the ground. I was eager to open the letters on my desk, but I had two babies at the hospital to examine and there was an emergency phone call coming in. The letters would have to wait until the end of the day.

The emergency call was from a Mr. Stallings, who was trying to decide whether the bat that had flown down his chimney this morning, and that he had bludgeoned to death with a broom, had been any threat to his four-month-old daughter. Many bats carry the rabies virus in their saliva, and rabies is a disease to be reckoned with.

After disposing of the bat in the garbage (I wish he had saved it, ideally chillled, for proper identification), as an afterthought, he decided to check on his baby daughter. To his horror, he noticed a fleck of blood on her ear. He asked me what he should do, but I told him I could not advise him properly without examining the baby. It was agreed that I would see the baby at the end of the day.

With morning hours concluded, two hours remained until I started afternoon appointments. Just enough time to examine the newborn babies and talk to their mothers.

On the way over to the hospital I was recalling how traumatic it was in the early years of our practice to vaccinate a child against rabies. It demanded fourteen days of inoculation with a duck egg vaccine that had to be administered beneath the skin of the abdomen. It was very painful for the child, an event that I am sure was never forgotten. Contemplating doing such a procedure on a small infant would have been an ordeal for all concerned. Fortunately, we have, in recent years, a new procedure that consists of five inoculations of a human diploid cell vaccine administered in the arm. It is much less traumatic and more protective. I snapped out of my reverie just about the same time I pulled into the hospital parking lot. Fortunately, the two babies I had to see were at the same hospital, which meant I would get back to the office in time to look at the letters waiting on my desk.

It was really a rather amusing visit. Mrs. Sanchez had just given birth to her fourth boy and Mrs. Mauer had just given birth to her fourth girl. They both gave me a knowing smile when I mentioned it to them. I know them well, so it did not surprise me when they both replied, using about the same words, "I wouldn't have it any other way, Doctor."

After completing my work at the hospital, I returned to the office where the rest of the day passed uneventfully.

Only one patient remained to be seen; the four-month-old baby with the possible bat bite. Then I would finally be able to open the solicitation response letters. I could hardly wait to get at them.

The solution to the four-month-old baby's bloody ear proved rather simple. Examination revealed a small linear scratch on the lobe of her right ear and some clotted blood under her right middle finger nail. No rabies, just a self-inflicted scratch. Mr. Stallings and I were equally relieved.

Now for those letters. There were five of them that our secretary had neatly placed on my desk, one on top of the other. I inspected each envelope before opening it, and realized that two of them were returned unopened and stamped, "Unable to deliver, no longer at this address."

Pushing them aside, I opened the others. The first letter was from a dear woman in Florida who was very active in organizing the Living Rosary in her parish after I had sent her the instructions on how to proceed. She sent me a nice donation for the poor and remarked in her letter that, "We have 150 members in Saint Gregory's parish Living Rosary. Also, I started the Living Rosary in two other parishes in our area.

"A friend of one of our members started the Living Rosary in her parish about 100 miles from Toronto. Another member of our Living Rosary moved to England and she started it in her parish there. So gradually you can see how it is spreading."

The second letter was from a woman who is practically a neighbor and contained a very generous donation. She said, "I was deeply touched by your letter and the formation of your new CPR Corporation. The stories and pictures of the terrible human suffering in

Africa are heartbreaking. I trust and pray that Our Lady will see that your aid reaches its destination. I am praying for the successes of your mission."

The third and final letter was wrapped in pure love. It was from a very poor widow with only a very meager Social Security income, but despite her own want, she sent me one tenth of her monthly income. She said, "I don't like to see people go hungry. I live in my old home and thank God for each day He allows me to live here. I'm close enough to walk to daily Mass, another blessing I enjoy. I do pray for the poor and suffering and hope this helps a little. I have been faithful to the Living Rosary and I would like you to know how my prayers were answered. My oldest brother was away from the Faith for many years and very bitter. Thank God and Our Blessed Mother he came back to the Faith and received last Sacraments.

"I also prayed for my oldest nephew, who fell away from the Faith. He was a heavy drinker. He was sick four days, and during that time he went to confession and received the last Sacraments and had a Catholic funeral.

"I had two lady friends who came back after being away from the Faith for many years. I still have several grandchildren who seem to have lost the Faith, but I'll continue to pray as long as I live."

This elderly woman's offering preached a sermon to me that I have not forgotten. Look at what her faithfulness to Christ through her constant prayers, generosity, and patience had won for her: a realization and appreciation of God's blessings and the knowledge that friends and close relatives separated from Christ were now united with Him forever. What more could any of us ever wish for on this earth for ourselves and all our loved ones, than to be united with Christ, His Mother and saints forever in Paradise.

Praise the widow's mite!

— 18 —

Rome

"Senore Evers, this is the Vatican calling."

"It's not possible," I thought to myself. I knew Jean and I wished for an audience with the Holy Father, but because of unforeseen circumstances, I had started procedures for such an audience much later than advisable.

"Are you there, Senore Evers?"

"Yes, yes," I anxiously replied.

"Please appear with your wife tomorrow morning, 6:30 AM, at the Porta de Bronze. You are to attend a private Mass celebrated by the Holy Father."

"Holy smokes," I thought to myself. We are actually going to see the Holy Father! I couldn't believe it.

I blurted, "What is the Porta de Bronze, please?"

Somewhat unbelievingly the caller replied, "It's the large bronze door in front of the right colonnade."

My next question was even more incredulous to the operator than the previous one. "I am sorry, but what is a colonnade?"

"You have never heard of a colonnade? Have you ever been to St. Peters before?"

"No, it's our first trip to Rome and we have yet to visit the Basilica." I'm sure by now she was wondering what kind of hayseed was seeking this audience.

Very tactfully she answered, "I am sure you will have no trouble, sir. The colonnades are the many spaced large columns to the right and the left of the Basilica. When you arrive, ask others who will be there. I am sure you will have no difficulty."

"We'll be there," I replied.

Turning to Jean I said, "You'll never believe it, but we have an audience with the Holy Father tomorrow."

My fantasy world started working. Would it be a private audience, just Jean, me, and the Holy Father? Having never experienced an audience, I didn't know what to expect. I had heard that every Wednesday the Pope has a huge audience with thousands of people assembled in St. Peter's Piazza. At this time he delivers an important spiritual message to those present which is meant for the world.

Other audiences are granted to a smaller, but yet very large, number of people and are held indoors in an auditorium. About a thousand people are invited to this type audience and unless you would get a front row seat, it is unlikely you would obtain a chance to meet him or even see him very well. This audience did not sound anything like the ones I had heard about.

The audience came to fruition through a continuing correspondence I had been carrying on with a humble Italian Missionary in Kenya, Africa, named Fr. Colussi Oswald. I had told him of our intention of visiting Rome. It was just news on my part, nothing more. He replied to my letter with much enthusiasm and said, "You must see the Pope, I insist upon it." In the letter, which was typed with a partially broken-down typewriter, he gave me a letter of introduction to the Pope's secretary, whom he knew personally, and likewise told me I must obtain a letter from our own Bishop. Fr. Oswald's letter had arrived about a month before our departure.

The day following the arrival of Fr. Oswald's letter, I called the Diocesan Chancery office and requested a letter of introduction. The Bishop's secretary replied, "Oh, I'm sorry Dr. Evers, but that will be quite impossible. These procedures take a minimum of six weeks."

Quite disheartened over the news, I told Jean that our chances of an audience had just evaporated. She replied, "Don't give up so easily. Why not ask one of the priests over at our Parish to write you a letter of recommendation and send that with Fr. Oswald's letter and we will see what happens. What do you have to lose?"

She was right, of course. Bless my optimistic bride. On receiving the letter of recommendation from our assistant pastor, I fired off both letters a few days short of our departure date.

I have always had the desire to actually shake hands or kiss the Papal ring of the "Vicar of Christ," but never believed it would happen. However, for those who aspire to the practice of "Spiritual Childhood" they should expect anything and everything from their generous Father, God. My journey is one of continuous learning. I had particularly wished to see the Holy Father because of my interest over the last two years in the medical diagnosis of "brain death." While serving on our Pediatric Intensive Care Committee to plan a protocol on diagnosing "brain death" in children, I started to become concerned about the exactness of the science employed in making this diagnosis. The reason for this stems from the fact that once the diagnosis is established, the law permits removal of organs for transplantation into people who are in need of them. The more I studied the issue, the more I became convinced that the medical community had no absolute means for determining the precise moment of death in a "brain dead" individual and that insoluble doubt remained as to whether the immortal soul, i.e., the vital principle responsible for life, had departed from the body. The letter I sent to Monsignor Stanislaw Dziwisz, the Papal secretary, explains it quite well:

Monsignor Stanislaw Dziwisz
Secretaria Personale Sua Santitia
Vaticano
Italia

September 21, 1990

Dear Monsignor Dziwisz,

On Thursday, December 14, 1989, the Holy Father addressed the participants in a congress on the determination of the moment of death, which was sponsored by the Pontifical Academy of Sciences. The congress was specifically interested in "brain death" and organ transplantation. In his address, the Holy Father reminded those present that "Scientists, analysts, and scholars must pursue their research and studies in order to determine as precisely as possible the exact moment and the indisputable signs of death." Because, as he said, "There is a real possibility that the life whose continuation is made unsustainable by the removal of a vital organ may be that of a living person, whereas the respect due to human life absolutely prohibits the direct and positive sacrifice of that life, even though it may be for the benefit of another human being who might be felt to be entitled to preference."

If it is possible that I could see the Holy Father I would like to present him with a scientific paper that I and a colleague of mine, Dr. Paul Byrne, have written on the subject of "brain death." It has just recently been accepted for publication in *Pharos*, a medical journal in the United States. It is our contention that no scientific medical way exists that can determine the precise moment of death and we believe that our paper clearly demonstrates this. We believe also that insoluble doubt exists as to whether the immortal soul has departed from the body and that vital organ transplantation should not be permitted when this doubt exists.

I read from an excerpt from the book, *Do Not Be Afraid* by Andre Frossard, that the Holy Father's consecration to the Blessed Mother's Immaculate Heart, using the formula of St. Louis de Montfort, was a turning point in his life. Reading this thrilled me, for the identical thing occurred to me when I consecrated myself to the Immaculate Heart of Mary using the formula of St. Louis de Montfort along with the thirty-three day preparation period. It changed my life.

My wife and I will be leaving the United States on the 11th of October, will spend four days in Yugoslavia, then arrive in Rome the 16th of October and depart the 24th. We will be staying at the Hotel Raphael, Largo Febo 2.

Sincerely in Jesus and Mary,
Dr. Joseph C. Evers

I remarked to Jean concerning my fantasy about a private audience. Jean has the gift of wisdom. "Honey, I doubt very much if we will have a private audience; you know what an important person the Pope is and how limited his time must be. I am sure there will be many other people there." I wasn't convinced and spent a sleepless night.

It was still dark when we arrived by taxi the next morning at St. Peter's Piazza. The massive Basilica was shrouded in morning mist. Departing from the taxi, we slowly made our way toward what we believed would be the right colonnade. The first rays of morning light appeared about the same instant that we spotted a very large and impressive twenty-five foot high bronze door at the end of what indeed was the right colonnade. As we approached the steps leading up to the door I noticed we were the only ones there. My heart jumped. It jumped again as the huge doors creaked open and two Papal guards, smartly attired in Renaissance garb, appeared. One stood at attention to the right of the door and the other was standing in the center peering out into the evaporating darkness.

About five minutes after our arrival another taxi came to a stop a short distance from us and deposited three more people: a priest and, as we would later find out, a couple from Allentown, PA. They also were the recipients of a Papal invitation. My fantasy of a private audience vanished with their appearance. We made brief introductions and made our way up the mysterious yet beckoning entrance.

As we approached the top step, the center guard stepped aside to make way for a young man dressed in a dark suit. He had a paper in his hand and he scanned it as he asked our names. With a welcoming smile he acknowledged us and then waved us inside, where we were immediately directed into a small waiting room.

An older man told us that as soon as all those invited arrived, we would leave for the Pope's private chapel. Very soon after he had spoken, about 40 recently ordained young priests entered the room. The older man, who was to prove to be our guide, checked off the names of all the priests on a list that he had and then asked us to follow him.

Our hearts quickened as we all moved out of the small room in which we were assembled. Only the click of heels resonating against the marble floor was heard as we briskly walked down a very long and relatively wide hallway.

An ancient, ornate marbled stairway curving its way heavenward, graced the end of the hallway. Faithfully following our guide we ascended two flights of stairs and then entered an elevator. After a brief ride up of one floor, we exited into an open courtyard, traversed it, and after going through a few other doors, we were ushered into a spacious room dominated at one end by a massive table and a large chair.

A small, thin priest with graying hair and a kindly face greeted us and introduced himself as Fr. Stanislaw, the Papal secretary. I don't know whether it was wishful thinking or not, but when I told him our names I imagined a hint of recognition. He told us that we would be attending the Holy Father's private daily Mass in just a few minutes. After Mas we would assemble in the same large room and personally meet the Holy Father. Excitedly, we followed him as he led us down a corridor of about 50 feet into the Pope's private Chapel. We slowly filed in, with Jean and I taking two seats in the rear of the Chapel. Under my arm I had tucked my paper on "brain death," which I still hoped to present to the Holy Father.

The Chapel, about 15 by 25 feet, was very beautiful. The floor was of white marble streaked with green. The walls were of white stone with stained glass windows. A large figure of the victorious resurrected Christ and a dove were woven into the dark green marbled ceiling. The altar was very simple in appearance, with the tabernacle directly behind it. To the right of the altar was a three-foot brown stone bas relief of St. Peter's crucifixion. To the left was another three-foot brown stone bas relief of the burial of Christ. However, the image that we all singularly and uniquely experienced was that of the Holy Father kneeling in deep meditation before the altar. So deep was he in prayer that he was unaware of our entrance.

It was a moment difficult to describe. All I can say is that I experienced this profound sense of being in the presence of a very holy and humble man. In radiating his own personal awareness of the presence of God, God became alive and present to us through the Holy Father at that moment. He communicated to us his own sense of "spiritual childhood" in the presence of the Almighty yet Loving God.

The Mass, said in Italian, was moving as it was beautiful, and receiving Jesus from the Pope's hands was a special joy to us all.

After the conclusion of Mass we assembled in the spacious greeting room outside the chapel. Monsignor Stanislow arranged each group in clusters of two to six around the periphery of the end of the room opposite to the table and chair. Jean and I formed one of the small groups. The Pope then entered and with his face glowing with love and kindness, he very slowly made his way around the room talking to each group. You could see his special fondness for the young priests as he engaged in short, friendly banter with them.

I could sense as he neared us that this was not the proper setting to be handing the Holy Father my paper on "brain death." I whispered some brief remark to Jean about it and she seconded the motion.

Finally the moment arrived. Monsignor Stanislaw spoke, "Your Holiness, this is Doctor and Mrs. Evers from McLean, Virginia."

The Holy Father repeated our name and we exchanged greetings. I extended my hand to shake his, but only afterwards realized that I should have kissed his ring. In his hand he held two Blessed Rosaries. He gave the first to Jean and the second to me.. After this he said words that I shall treasure all my life, "I give my blessing to you both and to the Evers family."

A photographer took a number of photos of each group so that each of us has a beautiful memento of our visit. As the Holy Father departed, Monsignor Stanislaw was about five feet behind him and at that moment I managed to get into the hands of the monsignor my article on "brain death." He gratefully received it and gave me the impression that he would give it to the Holy Father.

The audience with the Holy Father was the highlight of our visit to Rome. The rest of the visit, to the Colosseum, the Roman Forum, even St. John Lateran and the Vatican library, were all enjoyable, but were anti-climatic and eclipsed by the Papal visit.

We took many pictures while in Rome, one of which proved to have very interesting results. On our last day there we climbed the Aventine Hill to take a look through the famous keyhole on the large dark green doors guarding the entrance to the Knights of Malta. Looking through the keyhole, the tourist can see at the end of a narrow path framed by popular trees, the Basilica of St. Peters.

The Knights of Malta was founded in 1120 as a hospice and infirmary for pilgrims by Blessed Gerard and is dedicated to St. John the Baptist. At present the Order is a religious community of lay brothers and chaplains whose aim is the sanctification of its members through service to the faithful, the Holy See and in particular to the sick and the poor.

After a rugged climb to the top of the hill we found the Malta Palace, and after each one of us looked through the keyhole viewing St. Peters I took a chance at taking a picture. Holding the window of my camera against the keyhole, I snapped what was to be our last film on the role. As I said, the result of this picture was most intriguing.

After getting home I took the rolls of film to the drug store for developing and a few days later picked up the 3x5 pictures. Thirty minutes later Jean and I were reviewing our Roman journey. Coming to the keyhole picture, we gasped at the surprising results. The film turned out perfect in every respect. The keyhole was well outlined and through it was the narrow path bordered with the tall popular trees. However, instead of there being at the end of the path the Basilica of St. Peter's, in its place was a stream of ethereal light pouring through the end of the path. It was both mystifying and beautiful, and I did not know quite what to make of it.

The trip was in October, and that Christmas I decided to make a collage of our trip to Rome of the Papal visit and give it to Jean as a Christmas present. I bought a relatively large recessed display case, the back of which was lined with blue felt.

The focal point of the display was a picture of the Holy Father praying in deep meditation just before Mass. Jean and I can be seen in the last row. Above and below this picture were projecting supports on which I mounted a rock and some keys. The symbolism was obvious.

Beside the picture of the Holy Father I placed to its right the keyhole of Malta with the mysterious ethereal light. On the other side I placed another surprising picture. I had wanted to get some more copies of the keyhole picture, so I took the negative to a photographic shop and asked for another positive. Imagine my surprise when I picked up the photograph and found a perfect picture once again of the keyhole, the narrow path line by popular trees, but this time at the end of the path was not the ethereal light, but a perfect picture of St. Peter's Dome. How the same negative could give two different positive prints I cannot explain. But I placed this picture on the other side of the central picture of the Holy Father.

Jean and I had different interpretations of the ethereal light. She saw it as representing the holiness of John Paul the II. I saw it as the light of "St. Peter" shining in the darkness of our world and in transcending time and space, illuminating the narrow path to eternal life.

The collage captured the Gospel verse perfectly: "Thou art Peter, and upon this rock I will build My Church and the gates of Hell shall not prevail against it. And I will give thee the keys of the kingdom of heaven, and whatever thou shalt bind on Earth shall be bound in Heaven, and whatever thou shalt loose on Earth shall be loosened in Heaven."

John Paul II...what a treasure this Pope is to the Catholic Church. He, the Fatima Pope, having consecrated himself to the Immaculate Heart of Mary, is now that one voice crying out in the darkness of the error that so permeates our Church today.

By word and example he leads all those little ones, consecrated to the Immaculate Heart of Mary, down the path of prayer, penance, and daily mortification into the safe harbor of the Sacred Heart of Jesus. If the truth which he proclaims was only listened to and believed by all members of the clergy and laity of our age, it would effectively erase the present day apostasy.

Oh yes, Jean said she liked her Christmas present.

— 19 —

Jamaica

The most impressive sight about the interior of St. Jude's Church is the large wooden cross that hangs above and behind the main altar. It is easily six feet in height and on it hangs a wooden corpus of Christ. The face and body are roughly carved and from afar the features on the face look intimidating. A person may look at it and imagine our Saviour saying, "Look at what your sins have done to Me." It was the first time I had attended St. Jude's, and I must confess to an initial uneasiness upon viewing the face on the cross.

It was our first day in Jamaica and our second trip to work in Fr. Richard Albert's Medical Clinic. Jean and I were fortunate that year in having the company of our youngest daughter, Tara.

Jean decided to stay at the hotel and unpack, so she did not accompany Tara and me to Mass. As Fr. Albert vested for Mass and thirty or so Jamaican parishioners slowly filled the pews, my mind wandered to the events of the past year and a half leading up to this moment.

Our parish, St. Luke's, through its Outreach program to those in need, adopted St. Patrick's Catholic Church, a very poor parish located just outside Kingston Jamaica. One of our parishioners, who was a personal friend of Fr. Richard, introduced him to our Pastor, Fr. Steven Culkin. Both these men share a mutual concern for God's poor and their many needs. Within a short space of time this mutual concern gave birth to a linkage of love between our wealthy parish and Fr. Richard's poor parish.

Fr. Richard is a man worth meeting. His portly frame and short stature mask his boundless energy. Pastor of two parishes, St.

Patrick's and St. Jude's, founder of St. Elizabeth's home for the aged and lepers and also founder of Riverton Health Clinic and a newer medical facility just finished, St. Margaret's, he is a man in constant motion who exudes enthusiasm wherever he may be.

In the year and a half that our parish has had the privilege to be associated with St. Patrick's and Fr. Richard, several of our parishioners have gone down to Jamaica and have volunteered their time in the construction of new housing and in administering medical assistance to the poor.

The first medical clinic established by Fr. Richard was in Riverton City, where 5000 men, women, and children live in a dump on the edge of the city of Kingston. The poverty is heart-wrenching.

Well do I recall the first time Jean and I saw Riverton City. It was on our first trip to Jamaica and we were being chauffeured over to the medical clinic on a dirt road that twisted past a maze of shacks with rusted tin roofs and rotting lumber. Our driver had to be careful not to hit the half-naked, emaciated children wandering across our van's path. Poverty and filth were everywhere. It was unbelievable that people could live in such an environment.

Every now and then in the ten-minute drive through Riverton to the medical clinic, hope emerged in the form of brightly painted, well-constructed one-room homes. This was the product of Fr. Richard's efforts coupled with the young parishioners belonging to St. Luke's Outreach program who had journeyed to Jamaica to build these homes.

Our two successive mornings in Riverton went well. The clinic was nothing more than a six-by-twelve-foot concrete building that was divided in half. One half served as the waiting room for the patients, the other as the examination and treatment room. Because there was no running water at the clinic, all water used for compounding antibiotic prescriptions and washing hands had to be carried to the clinic.

Jean and I saw approximately 80 men, women, and children over the two-day period. One young man had symptoms of diabetes which I confirmed by doing a sugar test on his urine. I then referred him to the nearby hospital for insulin dosage and dietary instructions. Another small boy, about five years of age, was half blind. I referred him to an ophthalmologist and hoped he could be helped.

Reflecting on the events of our first journey to Jamaica and sitting in the pew waiting for Mass to start, I wondered what would happen during our present trip.

Perspiring profusely as he finished vesting for Mass, Fr. Richard removed his thick glasses to mop his face, brow, and balding head. The entrance hymn began as he walked to the altar to begin Mass. Once again the mystery of God's love unfolded in the reenactment of the unbloody sacrifice of our dear Saviour on Calvary's hill.

Fr. Richard's homilies are usually very good, and tonight's was no exception. I was glad Tara was there for the portion of the sermon I liked best.

"I want to tell you about a very special lady," boomed Fr. Richard in his rich baritone voice. "Her name is Lady Jane. I have known her for many, many years and slowly over this period of time she has lost, one by one, all her fingers and toes to the leprosy that has been slowly eating her body. Whenever I have the occasion to see her she almost invariably repeats the same message and the message is, 'Fr. Richard, I am the most blessed woman on the face of this earth. My sweet Jesus has saved me for His very own by shedding His precious Blood for me and my sins. I love Him so much.'

"How can anyone complain, my dear friends," said Fr. Richard, "after five minutes with this saintly woman. What a shining jewel she must be in the eyes of God."

I could tell by the look on Tara's face that she was deeply moved by Father's words.

Finishing the homily, Father motioned for us all to come up front and gather around the altar. I do not recall the exact moment that my eyes were directed once again to the cross over the altar. It was either at the Offertory or at the Consecration when Fr. Richard called our Saviour to St. Jude's altar. Nonetheless, a beautiful surprise met my eyes as I gazed up at the figure of Christ, a surprise that warmed my heart for the rest of the trip. Gone was the intimidating look which was actually nothing more than a mirage, for now up close, carved in the wood, there was a distinct and unmistakable smile on the face of our dying Saviour. Whether the original impression was an optical illusion from afar or the artist's intent, I do not know nor did it matter, for now our blessed Lord seemed to be saying, "Yes, it is I, your loving Saviour smiling in My suffering, so happy am I to save you, My little ones. For it is only when you are little, trusting and abandoned that you are able come close to Me and then viewing My smile you are able to perceive My intense love for all those of you who are My little children."

As it evolved, our second trip to Jamaica would prove to be as enjoyable and spiritually enriching as our first journey. Jean, Tara, and I would be the first medical team to work in the new medical facility at St. Margaret's.

St. Margaret's, an oasis of love made possible to Fr. Richard through a grant from the Netherlands government, is composed of several buildings located not too far down the road from St. Patrick's Church and school grounds. It not only has a pleasant two-room medical clinic, but also an adjoining office for Father. In addition it has a sewing room to teach young girls how to sew, and a woodworking room in which young men can be taught basic woodworking skills so that benches, planters, etc., can be built and sold. There is also a library and a room where children can find a safe place to study and be tutored. The library was made possible through the generous donation of the parishioners at St. Luke's. St. Margaret's is also providing a place where the elderly can come together and socialize and work on arts and crafts as well as interact with the young children when appropriate. Finally, St. Margaret's provides a place where young pregnant teenagers can continue their education and have baby care facilities if necessary.

On our first day there Fr. Richard introduced us to Nurse Burkes, an Irish nurse who volunteers her help in the clinics four days a week. Her knowledge and expertise were most helpful, and we valued her presence. There was also a native Jamaican doctor, whom we did not meet, who occasionally saw patients on a Saturday morning at the Riverton facility.

Tara worked as our receptionist, greeting the patients and giving them a number signifying their turn. Jean and Nurse Burkes provided nursing and pharmaceutical care. The only drugs prescribed had to be available on the shelf in the medical examining rooms where we worked. As I examined each patient and prescribed the proper medication, the nurse would take the medication from the shelf and count out either the correct number of pills or pour into a container, brought by the patient, a prescribed liquid medication. In all we saw about one hundred patients, most of whom were children.

I had quite a few interesting and unfortunately sad cases. One particularly sad case was when, at St. Margarets, a mother brought in a little two and a half-year-old girl who was partially paralyzed. She was unable to stand and had to get about by crawling on her knees, dragging her legs and feet after her. I wish there was something we could have done to help her, and I know if she had been in America, physical medicine and proper bracing could have been of help. I was not sure what her diagnosis was; infantile paralysis was a possibility.

A somewhat humorous yet sad situation evolved when a mother brought her five children in for various illnesses. Two of the children were twin four-year-old boys with pot bellies. Harold had a very serious look to his face and Winston, the other boy, a happy grin. Their mother told me they ate dirt all the time and wondered if this was contributing to their pot bellies. I noticed that they had sway backs which pushed their bellies out. I said, "Mother, they have sway backs, and that is the reason their stomachs are sticking out." I added, "I have sway back myself and my stomach sticks out." She smiled and then asked me, "What are you going to do to make them stop eating dirt, Doctor?" I really didn't have the foggiest idea what I was going to do and I didn't have any handy reference. The only thing I could think of was instant psychotherapy. I took the boy with the serious face and, putting my hands over his cheeks, I tilted his head up so his eyes met mine and said in a very firm voice, "Harold, you are never, never, to eat dirt again. Do you understand?" Wide eyed, he kept nodding in agreement with my adamant recommendation. With Winston the same command was repeated, firmer than ever. Holding his head in the same manner, I asked Winston what he was going to do, and with that same grin he replied, "I am never, never, going to eat dirt again." I knew that with all that dirt they had ingested there was a chance that a few worms had also been eaten. Therefore, I prescribed to each of them some worm medicine. Only time will tell whether I helped them.

The most satisfying case was that of a ten-year-old little girl who was brought in by her mother because she was acting "crazy" at school. After a laborious history-taking session with the mother that both my wife and I struggled with for some time due to a language difficulty, we finally realized the child was having grandmal seizures. Through Nurse Burke's efforts, she will be seen by a Jamaican neurologist and the proper anti-convulsant medication will be prescribed. The majority of the patients were ailing from those diseases that we all seek comfort and relief from, bronchitis, throat infections, colds, stomach aches and with the little ones, ear infections.

Fr. Albert asks that each family pay the equivalent of twenty-five cents for the office visit. In this way each person is able to maintain their sense of self-worth and dignity.

We are not the only ones who have had the privilege of going to Jamaica to work in Fr. Albert's medical clinic. Another St. Luke's parishioner family, Dr. Bill Byrnes, his wife Mary, and their daughter Dedee and son John have gone down the last two years. Bill is a thoracic surgeon, Dedee a family practitioner now studying to be a surgeon, and John an orthopedic surgeon.

I do not know how many Catholic Parishes throughout the United States are involved in the same type of outreach program of helping very poor parishes at home and abroad, but it indeed is a viable way to give life to St. Francis's prayer:

"O Divine Master, grant that I may not so much seek to be consoled as to console, to be understood as to understand, to be loved as to love, for it is in giving that we receive, it is in pardoning that we are pardoned, it is in dying [to self] that we are born to eternal life."

We all agreed that going to Jamaica was a very special blessing given to us by the Lord because through Him we carry His love and compassion to the poor who, as the Bible clearly states, are His favorites.

— 20 —

The Gift

Jean, the children and I were visiting my parents and I had decided to accompany my mother to the 7:00 AM weekday Mass. We had arrived early at Saint Pius the Tenth's church and were leisurely walking up the side steps when suddenly I noticed, about 100 feet above the ground, flying in perfect V formation, a squadron of mallards. My eyes were fixed on them, admiring the beauty and precision of their flight, when three of the birds from the rear of the formation peeled off and, diving low over the Church dome, dipped their wings in salute.

Even nature responds in awe and reverence over God's gift to humanity, for directly beneath the church dome the Blessed Sacrament is kept in a spacious marble tabernacle on St. Pius the Tenth's high altar.

As long as I can remember I have been blessed with a lively faith in the true presence of Jesus Christ in the Blessed Sacrament. I owe the seeds of this faith to my parents. I recall when I was a five year old youngster, my mother pointed out to me in our local parish church the tabernacle and told me, "Joe, Jesus lives in there."

This declaration of faith, repeated over and over, made a profound impression on me. My favorite spot in church was the front pew. During Mass, every time the priest opened the tabernacle door, I would stretch my neck and strain my eyes in hopes of catching a glimpse of baby Jesus inside the tabernacle. My mother had showed me pictures of the Infant Jesus dressed as the Infant of Prague, and I fully expected through my five-year-old eyes to see Infant Jesus inside His little house, richly adorned in the Infant of Prague garments.

My faith in Christ's presence in the Blessed Sacrament has never diminished over the years, but has only steadily increased. I thank God for this grace, for it is truly just that, a grace from God.

About fifteen years ago I received a special blessing with the privilege of being permitted to function as a Eucharistic minister in our own parish.

There were two home-bound parishioners that particularly stand out in my mind; I had the unique joy of bringing frequently to their bedside our sweet Saviour. One individual was an old man by the name of Joe. He had a hearing aid and it was difficult to perform the short ceremony of prayers surrounding the reception of the Eucharist because I had to shout in his ear. Nonetheless, we managed to get through the prayer service and Joe, with great devotion, would receive his dear Saviour. The manner in which he received the Sacrament was very edifying and a source of great spiritual benefit for myself, for more than a few times I saw tears running down Joe's cheeks during his Communion thanksgiving.

On the Feast of the Immaculate Conception, a few months before Joe died, I received a beautiful Eucharistic consolation. Joe was staying with his daughter and her family, and while driving up their winding driveway to their woods-hugged home I noticed, when some thirty yards from the front entrance, a large silhouetted Nativity scene, accented in green, atop the lattice outdoor entrance way. After administering Communion to Joe I told his daughter how attractive it was and inquired as to who had constructed it. I was surprised to hear she knew nothing about it. Upon leaving, imagine my delight when, upon examining the Nativity scene more thoroughly, I discovered that it was formed by several large green leaves that sprouted from a vine that covered the entrance way. At a distance from ten to thirty feet, it resembled to anyone's eyes a perfectly silhouetted Nativity Scene.

Oh yes, I almost forgot, Joe was summoned home to his sweet Saviour on his birthday. What a wonderful birthday present. Eternal life with Love!

On another occasion I had the great privilege of bringing our dear Saviour almost daily to a physician colleague friend of mine who was dying of cancer. His name was John; I recall him saying more than once, "Joe, you will never know how much peace and consolation I receive from Holy Communion."

At other times he would become morose and I would inquire why. He would answer, "Well Joe, it's a little scary facing death and all one must answer for to the Lord." I would then remind him of the Brown Scapular he wore and then he would smile and respond, "Oh yes, the Blessed Mother's protection is such a joy."

I thank this same Mother for another Eucharistic consolation I received. It occurred during the octave of the Assumption. It was a beautiful day, the sky was a deep blue with a few scattered clouds and the sun was at its zenith in the heavens. I had just left John's house and was standing in the driveway after giving him Communion and recalled that I had neglected to consume several particles of the Host that remained in the pyx. At the same moment I recalled this, I was inspired to reverence the particles of the Sacred Host before consuming them. After reverencing them, I was thrilled when I opened the pyx and saw that the particles were perfectly arranged in a pattern resembling the Infant of Prague. The brilliant August sunshine sparkling on the inner surface of the pyx intensified this beautiful and meaningful personal event.

These two consolations and serving as Eucharistic minister deepened my faith in the true presence of our Saviour in the Blessed Sacrament. For a number of years I have made it a practice to make a weekly Holy Hour, and for a time I was able to do this daily. I consider this one of the greatest privileges we poor sinners can have on earth.

I am concerned that in these present times there exists a certain undesirable dampening in the reverence and awe that should be present in our hearts for this great gift, the Eucharist. Witness the fact that a certain number of parishioners fail to genuflect in the presence of the Blessed Sacrament before entering the pew. Such disrespect was unthinkable less than thirty years ago. Witness also the fact that the King of Kings is in more than a few parishes placed in a tabernacle on a side altar or is not even in the main body of the Church at all, being relegated to a private chapel that is rarely visited.

No longer in many parishes are there the customary wonderful forty hour devotions that we had in bygone years. On feasts dedicated to the Eucharist, gone is the majestic procession of the Blessed Sacrament with the priest in rich vestments carrying the monstrance.

However, by no means am I disheartened, for in certain parishes I have observed a springtime Eucharistic renewal. One parish in our community has perpetual adoration of the Blessed Sacrament and at any hour the faithful can be found in prayer. Not long ago I was making my customary Holy Hour in this church when a grandmother with her four-year-old grandson briefly came into the adoration chapel. It was a joy to hear the conversation between them. "That's Jesus," said his grandmother, and the little boy unabashedly replied while waving his hand in the direction of the monstrance harboring the Sacred Host, "Hello Jesus, hello Jesus."

"Tell Jesus you love Him," added the grandmother.

The little fellow then echoed, "I love You, Jesus, I love You."

No greater catechism lesson in the true presence was possible than the one I had witnessed that day.

In a nearby parish where I frequently make a visit to the Blessed Sacrament I am struck by the genuine reverential teaching given the school children by the nuns and teachers in respect for the Eucharist. In our own parish there are plans to have a weekly Holy Hour for any of the parishioners who wish to attend. These happenings, I believe, are favorable signs.

The greatest form of prayer that we Catholics can participate in is the Holy Sacrifice of the Mass. The Daily Mass League Pamphlet published by Pro Trinitas states, "One Mass gives God more praise and thanksgiving, makes more atonement for sin, and pleads more eloquently than does the combined eternal worship of all the souls in Heaven, on earth, and in Purgatory. In the Holy Mass, it is Jesus Christ, God, as well as Man, who is our Intercessor, our Priest and our Victim. Being God as well as Man, His prayers, merits, and His sufferings are infinite in value."

I have witnessed the power of the Mass in its ability to heal, reconcile, and convert. My greatest recent memories center around the "Healing Mass." Just in the past few years that I have been promoting it through the CPR Corporation, people are being healed of crippling anxieties, mental depression, and scrupulosity. Still others are reporting modest economic help, marital strengthening, and a return to the Sacrament of reconciliation of someone in their family.

Not too long ago, I received a call from a friend of mine whose 25-year-old daughter has attempted suicide twice. She has been paralyzed from the waist down since seven years of age and has never been able to resolve in her own mind this unfortunate accident. Approximately one month ago I had one of my missionaries offer a "Healing Mass" for her, their family, and their family tree. The father called me to tell me that since the "Healing Mass" a beautiful Christian couple has entered their daughter's life and they have taken an immense interest in her. She already is beginning to show signs of hope.

On another occasion a mother entered my office with her son and thanked me for the "Healing Mass" that one of my missionaries had offered for her, her family, and their family tree. This was made possible by her own mother who had mentioned to me that her daughter was in a mental institution, deeply depressed, and that she was in danger of losing her son to her estranged husband. Now the smiling young mother informed me that she had been released from the hospital and was on a new kind of medicine that was helping her a great deal. She has more hope now than she had had in a long time.

Last year a "Healing Mass" was offered for a friend of mine and her family. During the year her father and younger sister died. One does not ordinarily associate God's blessings with death. However, her father had been ill for some time and he died a beautiful Christian death. Having received the last Sacraments, he died clothed in the Scapular of Our Lady of Mount Carmel. His death was an occasion of family healing and reconciliation.

Her younger sister also suddenly became ill and after a short illness also died clothed in the Scapular of Carmel and with the last Sacraments of the Church. A wonderful added blessing was the discovery in her death the "jewel" of her life. My friend tells it best.

Handicapped No More

Our sister, Susan Kathleen, made the best of her handicapped earthly life. We never knew for sure whether Susan had Down's Syndrome or another syndrome that mentally impaired her. But what she lacked in IQ, she more than made up for in wisdom and love.

In July, 1989, Susan died only three-plus weeks after being diagnosed with cancer, the primary unknown. She died as she had lived, bravely and beautifully, despite agonizing symptoms. She felt sad about dying so unexpectedly and at only thirty-eight years of age; but she left loving messages for many and touched us all deeply in her living and in her dying.

Whatever handicaps she had in this life, she kept in touch with Our Lord and had accepted our Saviour into her heart. She is handicapped no more.

In talking to my friend, she tells me that her sister left a remarkable diary, unknown to all in her family, with instructions that it was not to be read until after her death. My friend is an author, so God's plan has yet to unfold in respect to Susan living and dying, a loving instrument in God's hands.

Through word of mouth and the Corporation I manage I inform people about the "Healing Mass," and if they are interested I give them the following information packet.

The Healing Mass

We all know the awesome power of Christ's redemptive sacrifice when His cleansing Blood was poured out for us on Calvary's Hill, but many of us fail to fully realize that each and every Mass offered is the same sacrifice as that of Calvary and has merited for us every grace that we might need.

There is not a family on the face of the earth that is not affected in some way or another with spiritual, physical, or psychological problems consequent to original and personal sin. This consequence to the sin of Adam has affected not only us, but our entire family tree, both ancestral and those yet to be born. However, we need not despair, but on the contrary should rejoice, for our Loving and Merciful Saviour offers us the opportunity to cleanse our entire family tree through His Eucharistic Sacrifice, the Holy Sacrifice of the Mass.

I obtained this knowledge from a book that I read on the subject by a well-known Charismatic priest where he stated in truth that "the Eucharist is the most powerful means known since the sin of Adam in healing the Family Tree."

I myself had a "Healing Mass" said for my entire Family Tree. Even though I was unable to attend the Mass in person, I did attend a Mass in another church 2000 miles distant on the day that this special Mass was being offered.

Before having the Mass said I prepared for it by building up my faith, through meditation, in the power of the Mass. In my preparation I meditated on Christ's mercy and love and also meditated on each one I was praying for. I made it a special point to forgive them for any wrong they may have been responsible for and in turn I asked their forgiveness. (When possible I either spoke to them or wrote to them about it.) I also sent a letter to the priest offering the Mass in which I listed my intentions and asked if he would place it on the altar the day he said the Mass. The results were dramatic. Someone, from whom I had been partially estranged since childhood, I now am closer to than ever before in my adult life. The Lord created circumstances shortly after the Mass was said which permitted this beautiful healing to occur. Also, a short time after the Mass was said a partial deeper healing of other concerns occurred. There still remain other intentions that have yet to be answered, but I am certain that in God's good time they will be. Praise God! Praise the precious Blood of our Saviour.

The CPR Corporation (a Corporation I founded to help the poor) corresponds with many missionaries in Africa and India, any of whom could say a "Healing Mass" for your Family Tree. A Healing Mass could be said for a cleansing of your entire family tree by and through the Sacred Blood of Christ.

When the Mass is said you should dwell not so much on the problems of the family, but on Jesus' mercy, love, and forgiveness. In order for the healing to be successful, there must be a genuine forgiveness on your part of all members of your family tree that have been hurt through sin of another. You should ask for a complete healing of all spiritual, psychological, and physical impairments.

God asks for effort on our part, but the reward is great. The better one prepares, the more faith one has, the better the results.

This is the address of a priest I know who lives in xxxxxxx who I am sure would help you if you cannot find anyone else.

I then write the address of the priest. If the person can afford it, I ask for a small donation to the CPR Corporation (tax-deductible) as a stipend for the priest offering the Mass and for the poor they serve. If they cannot afford it I will make the donation myself.

Not to be forgotten is the virtue of patience, because some intentions take longer than others to be answered. Jesus has His own agenda and always knows what is best for us.

God's love is so deep that it is unexplainable to us mortals. Infinite Love...who can comprehend it? His love brings us together, His love is responsible for every good inspiration and good action you or any of us have ever done. How fortunate we are to know Him and to be able to love and serve Him. Glory be to the Father, the Son, and the Holy Spirit! Now and forever, Amen!

— 21 —

The Little One

A light snow was falling and it was cold. It was the type of snowfall that would stick, and already three or four inches had accumulated. Snowflakes are like people: each one is unique. Incredible, isn't it? I recall as a child in my hometown, snowbound Buffalo, New York, running around outside catching snowflakes in my hand and then, with my other hand, examining them with a magnifying glass. I was fascinated and excited over the intricate yet beautiful pattern of each flake. If only they wouldn't melt so quickly. If only I could have permanently captured at least one of them and mounted it for display, like one mounts butterflies.

Our car was moving slowly toward the church following others. We came to an intersection just at the church entrance and I was concentrating on making the turn, so I didn't notice the hearse. Jean noticed. It had arrived at the intersection the same moment our car did. Mary Alice had died just three days ago, on Jean's birthday. It was a peaceful death; she had slipped into hepatic coma secondary to liver metastasis. It was as if she descended into a deep, deep sleep from which she never would awake.

A few days earlier at the wake I had been talking to Johnny, her younger brother. He strongly resembled Mary Alice, the same penetrating eyes, the same happy, sparkling smile. They just had to be brother and sister. He shared with me the last words that she spoke to him. He hadn't seen her in almost six months and had purchased some new glasses. He tells it better.

"Joe, it was the day before she went into the coma and all day she been drifting into and out of a deep sleep. I was bending

over her trying to get a response our of her. The nurse had just
finished fluffing up her pillow. I think I said something like, 'Mary
Alice, Mary Alice, it's Johnny. Can you hear me?' I had to repeat it
several times but finally I reached her; she groaned and then smiled."

"She was able to smile?" I incredulously replied.

"Well, you know Mary Alice. Yes, she smiled and then I barely
heard her say, 'Johnny, is that you?'"

"Yes, it's me," I replied, "how are you doing?"

"She then opened her eyes, looked at me and, ignoring my
question, weakly replied, 'Johnny, good to see you. Hey, I like your
glasses, they look really neat.'"

I saw a tear in Johnny's eyes as he told me the last words Mary
Alice ever spoke, not only to him, but to all of us. That was so
typical of Mary Alice; always thinking of others, even on her death
bed. No mention of her own pain, her own fears. She only knew
how to give, to give, and then to give some more.

A little over two years ago, George Flowers operated on her
for intestinal obstruction. He found no evidence of reoccurrence
and all those who loved her were very optimistic about the future.
She had returned to work in our office and was her old bouncy self.
The first hint of trouble was six months after her operation when,
while at the beach with her husband Tom, she noticed a sharp pain
in her lower right chest while opening a window. She thought it
was nothing more than a sprained muscle, but it continued to bother
her every time she took a deep breath. About two weeks after returning home she saw Charlie Masters, who was not only my own
personal physician, but Mary Alice's as well. X-rays were obtained
and in a brief telephone conversation with Charlie I recall him saying, "Nothing more than a cracked rib, Joe."

I replied, "Sounds like good news to me, Charlie. You say no
suspicious shadows on the film, that's great. From what I have read
about her particular tumor it rarely, if every, metastasizes to bone."

"Yeah, I think you're right, Joe," answered Charlie.

At the time, our appraisal of Mary Alice's condition made sense
to us. After all, she had undergone two major operations in the last
nine months and it was only natural that because her body was a
little run down a rib could easily crack. As for myself, I honestly
believed she was on the road to a complete recovery.

Unfortunately, my optimism lasted only a few weeks. No sooner had her first rib healed when another one snapped, and then another. I still refused to believe it was metastasis, but Charlie and others thought otherwise and insisted on a biopsy. How wrong I was. I was crushed when the biopsy report came back positive. We all were.

Poor Mary Alice. The disease was unrelenting. At approximately the same time the biopsy report had come back. It showed signs that the cancer had spread, and pain — together with a noticeable limp — had developed in her right hip. We knew the disease had now invaded her pelvis, and X-rays confirmed it.

Bone pain, particularly bone pain secondary to cancer metastasis, can be excruciating. Yet during her long illness I never saw Mary Alice cry but on one occasion. I vividly recall the occasion. It was about a year before her death and by then her whole spine had become involved. Fortunately, although limping badly, she was still able to walk. She and Tom were getting ready to go to a church service and it was while attempting to get out of a chair into a standing position that a wave of paralyzing pain, triggered by back spasms, spread throughout her whole body.

Tom telephoned me immediately and with obvious anxiety in his voice described the problem. "Joe, I don't know how to help her, she can't even move a muscle without crying out in pain."

"Any possibility of picking her up and carrying her into your bedroom?"

"No, she can't tolerate me even touching her."

Listening to Tom, I pictured Mary Alice frozen with pain in a grotesque posture. Pain...how does one measure it, how does one define it?

The worst pain I ever experienced was due to a kidney stone. I felt as though a horse was kicking me in the stomach. On a scale of one to ten, I would give kidney colic a six or a seven. Labor pains described by women who have also experienced kidney colic are even more intense. The most severe type of pain a person can experience is a form of neuralgia called tic doleroux. It's a chronic inflammation of the fifth facial nerve in which violent bursts of pain rhythmically spread over the face. So severe is it that patients suffering from this disorder have, while screaming in agony, fainted. If tic doleroux is a ten, Mary Alice was experiencing a solid nine.

"Tom, can't you give Mary Alice a morphine shot?"

While waiting for an answer, I could hear Mary Alice's distant, pleading voice asking her husband for help.

"Joe, Charlie just instructed me how to do it last week. I've been practicing with the needle and syringe on oranges, but haven't tried it on Mary Alice yet."

"Okay, look, tell Mary Alice to hang on, Tom. Jean and I will be right over."

The elapsed time travel from our house to theirs was usually about ten minutes. This evening we made it in eight. Not even bothering to knock or ring the bell, we burst inside the front door. Tom heard us enter and yelled, "Joe, Jean, in the downstairs bedroom."

Going directly to the bedroom, we entered and were surprised to see that Mary Alice had somehow made it to her bed and was now, like a rigid statue, laying flat on her back on the right side of the bed. A look of terror was in her eyes.

Surprised, I said, "How did you manage to make it to the bed?"

Tom, now on the stairs, answered. "The spasms stopped for a few moments and she was able to creep with my help over to the bed."

"Jeannie, Jeannie," Mary Alice was crying as she spoke to my wife. "It was terrible honey, I've never had pain like this in my life."

Tom, with a hypodermic syringe in his hand, said with a note of satisfaction, "I just gave my first shot."

"Good boy, Tom," I replied. "She should be getting some relief in a few moments."

Thankfully, the opiate worked quickly and Mary Alice fell into a fitful sleep. Tom would become an expert over the succeeding months in giving relief to his wife. Fortunately, she never quite experienced back spasms with the intensity that she had on that occasion, but her road to final peace continued to be paved with unrelenting pain.

I recall the October prior to her death that after office hours I used to go over to her house for a visit and then say a Rosary with her before leaving. Mary Alice was still able to hobble around some, but it was with great difficulty.

I remember on one particular visit her sufferings had increased and she was lying on the sofa for a bit of relief. I looked at her sensing her agony and said, "Mary Alice, you are a living cruci-fix." I know this sounds like a strange remark to make, but that was the only thought that came to mind at the moment. She looked at me a little surprised, and with a soft smile questionably replied, "Do you really think so?"

Looking at her I recalled John Paul II's wonderful encyclical entitled, "On the Christian Meaning of Human Suffering." In it he had reminded us that "Suffering seems to be, and is, almost in-separable from man's earthly existence," and that it must be faced because "the Redemption was accomplished through the Cross of Christ, that is through His suffering."

The Encyclical further reminds us that although suffering some-times is inflicted on man because of his sin, it is done for a purpose in order to "serve for conversion, that is, for the rebuilding of good-ness in the subject, who (hopefully) can recognize the divine mercy (of God's call) to repentance."

The one sentence that stood out for me in the Encyclical was the one that said, "Christ also becomes in a particular way united to the man (i.e. the man who accepts Christ) — through the Cross." In other words, when we sincerely and honestly accept our suffer-ing for the honor and glory of God in His continuing work of re-demption, we become intimately united with Jesus and His Cross.

Mary Alice was doing this, but she was so humble that she didn't even realize how fully she had embraced the cross, the cross of redemptive suffering.

The snow was coming down heavier and I wondered if the funeral cortege would have any difficulty en route to the grave site. I was standing in the church vestibule at the conclusion of Mass looking out the window. I could see that the pastor had instructed the grounds-keeper to plow the driveway. He was still working on it as Mary Alice's friends filed out of the church into their cars.

Mary Alice's dying, like her life, had its own particular mean-ing to each of us. I recalled the pastor's last words at the wake the night before. He is a fellow not given to soapy sentimentality, but he said it all when, with a noticeable crack in his voice, he con-cluded, "She had a smile that wouldn't quit."

Charlie, her physician, remarked to me sometime during her long illness, "You know, Joe, Mary Alice was the type of person I loved making a house call on. No matter how bad a day I had she would always cheer me up. Crazy, isn't it; the doctor is supposed to cheer the patient up. With Mary Alice it was different."

With my one hand on the wheel and my other interlocked in Jean's, we slowly and carefully followed the car in front of us. They were proceeding toward the cemetery extra carefully because of the snowfall. I was thinking about what Charlie had said concerning Mary Alice when I remarked to Jean, "What did you think of the final hymn?" It was my wife's favorite, a beautiful one entitled, "Do Not Be Afraid." I was surprised to hear it because I hadn't realized it must have been a favorite of Mary Alice's also. Jean didn't answer at first, but with a wane smile and slowly shaking her head to and fro she remarked, "I never heard her mention it." We both had the same thought simultaneously. Mary Alice knew that it was Jean's favorite hymn. It was just like her to mention to someone that she would want it sung at her funeral Mass.

As the procession of cars twisted and turned through the cemetery road, the tombs covered with snow resembled wingless angels standing at attention. As we neared the grave site, my mind wandered to a dinner meal Jean and I shared with Tom and Mary Alice quite some time ago. I recalled it as though it were yesterday, the whole delightful evening. We were seated at a corner table near the fire at our favorite restaurant. The glimmer of candlelight from the hurricane lamp reflected off Mary Alice's and Jean's faces. Many people who did not know them thought they were sisters. Even their voices were mistaken at times on the office telephone. Tom unfortunately had another one of his headaches, but was bearing up rather well. Jean, our oldest daughter Sharon, our youngest daughter Tara, and I had just returned from an eight day holiday on the tiny Caribbean island of Barbados. We had quite an adventure. I recall the conversation vividly.

I hate to fly and wish the Wright brothers had never tinkered around with air-frames, struts, and such. It was Mary Alice who, recalling my aerophobia, remarked, "Did ya like the airplane ride this time, Joe?" She laughed a hardy, teasing laugh and, turning her head to Jean said, "Were his knuckles white, Jeannie?"

Jean smile, "He's getting braver, Mary Alice They were just a mild blue this time."

Interrupting their sabered banter I said, "What are you talking about, I thought I did pretty good."

"Well, Mary Alice," Jean replied, "I have to admit that for a guy who gets airsick walking on a six-inch curb, he wasn't too bad this trip."

We all joined in the laughter, Tom enjoying it most of all.

It was a wonderful evening as my wife and I reviewed in delicious detail for our very good friends the various shops we visited, scenery we absorbed, and culinary cuisine we enjoyed. They love our girls and wanted to know their reaction to each experience. We were sipping our coffee when Mary Alice remarked, "But I thought you said you had an adventure. So far it sounds like another Evers junket."

"Well, Mary Alice," I replied, "I was saving the best for last."

"Oh," answered Tom, playfully raising his eyebrows, "what happened?"

"We got lost."

"Lost!" Tom gleefully howled, "How could you get lost on a postage stamp island?"

"It was like this, we spent the afternoon exploring the western end of the island going up one road and down the other. You know Jean."

Mary Alice understood what I was referring to, and shook her head in agreement. My wife loves exploring the unknown, the more remote and desolate, the better. I sort of enjoy it too. But the girls despise it and always fear the worst. This time they were right.

"Well anyway, the sun was starting to set and we were out on this peninsula. I felt as though we were in one of those English boxwood gardens, you know, one of those mazes from which there is only one exit. After winding around three times on this narrow two lane road and coming back to the same spot each time, the girls were getting more and more nervous, despite their mother's best efforts to bolster their sagging spirits. Finally, I spotted a mailbox on what I thought was a private road. Up the road was an old black man ambling along. Slowly driving up the road, I stopped the car right opposite him and explained our predicament. He was most helpful and told us to stay on this road which I thought was a private one. Sure enough, it got us back on the main drag just as the sun set."

Tom lit up a cigarette as Mary Alice enviously eyed his enjoyment. They both smoke, but only Tom in our presence. Mary Alice looked at me and said, "You really did have an adventure, didn't you?"

"This wasn't the end of it," replied Jean excitedly.

"You mean there is more?" Tom laughed. I noticed he hadn't said a word about his headache and presumably was feeling better. He usually screws up his face and almost unconsciously rubs his fingers over his eyes when it's bothering him. Our story must have taken his mind off it.

Jean laughingly continued, "The trip home is the good part. You wouldn't believe it Mary Alice, but the airplane was packed with tourists and there was a two-hour delay at one of the island stops on the way home. They forgot to serve us anything to eat until very late in the day. By the time we landed at New York City everybody was in a terrible mood. We sat on the tarmac another forty-five minutes before we left the airplane."

I caught the waiter's eye and motioned for another refill. Our little restaurant had great coffee and Mary Alice and I were hopeless addicts. While the waiter poured I jostled my wife's memory, "Tell them how much time we had, honey, to catch our connecting flight back home."

"Twenty minutes, that's all we had. Can you imagine just twenty minutes from the time we finally left the plane?"

"And," I interrupted, "we had immigration, customs, and a different airline to check in with."

"Well, Mary Alice, Tom," Jean's eyes flashed with excitement, "you can't imagine the next few minutes. We ran, I mean we literally ran, through the airport with Joe leading the way. It took us only a few minutes to find, and almost like magic, pass through immigration. We then headed for customs. You know how long it usually takes to get through customs."

"And at Kennedy airport," exclaimed Tom, "it has taken me hours."

"Well," continued Jean, "the customs line was long and it was packed with people and baggage, but as we approached the end of the line, out of nowhere a kind-faced, white-haired customs officer motioned for us to follow him."

"Yeah," I interrupted Jean again; I just couldn't resist telling this portion of the saga. "He looked at Jean and the rest of us and all he said was, 'I can tell you're trying to make a connecting flight, folks, do you have anything to declare?' We didn't, of course, and told him so. 'Right this way, then.' He let us into the main portion of the terminal. I was eyeing my watch all the while and saw we had eight minutes until our connecting flight left. I almost despaired, but Sharon, our eldest, rallied me on and said to us all, 'Let's run!' So we ran with Tara and Sharon leading the way. With shouts of 'This way, take a right,' and 'Take a left,' we skidded in this direction and dashed in that direction. With luggage flopping at our sides and sweat dripping from our faces, Jean and I started laughing at what a spectacle we must have made.

"With three minutes showing on my watch we finally found the right airline check-in-counter and once again out of nowhere stepped a kind-faced, courteous man with a tell-tale uniform on identifying him as an employee of our connecting airline. We felt as though he had been waiting for us since we left Barbados.

"'This way folks, this way. Just leave your luggage here, I'll take care of it.' Then briefly looking at our tickets, he pointed us in the right direction and swish, swish, after one last sprint before we knew it, we were in front of the boarding gate.

"I approached the woman behind the last barrier before we could ascend the boarding ramp and showed her our tickets. She shouted at another woman asking, 'Has 107 left yet? There are four more passengers.'

"The other woman answered, 'I think it may have, I'll check.'

"We all held our breath as she talked with an unheard and unseen voice on the phone. The thought of spending the night in Kennedy airport was unthinkable.

'No, the plane has not left yet, but they will have to open the door again.'

"'Okay folks,' said the first woman, 'hurry up please, you made it by only a few seconds.'

"We boarded the plane amid bewildered, inquisitive, and hostile stares from the passengers. We embarrassingly sought the four remaining seats and no sooner had strapped on our belts when the plane taxied for takeoff. The rest of the trip, except for the misplaced baggage, which finally caught up with us, was without surprises, but it was a trip we would not soon forget."

Grinning at Mary Alice I said, "I call that an adventure, wouldn't you, Mary Alice?"

"Yeah, yeah, that's an adventure!"

The evening over, we left in our car and headed for our friends' home. We always took only one car and on this particular evening it was our turn to drive. On the way home we continued to talk about our island adventure, reminiscing here, embellishing there. Just before reaching our friends' home, I became a little serious and said, "Honey, should I tell them about Fr. Dominic's sermon at Mass the day after we got home?"

"Oh, I almost forgot. Yes, tell them."

"The conclusion, eh?" said Mary Alice.

"Yes, the real conclusion, Mary Alice. Fr. Dominic, the assistant Pastor at our church, gives excellent sermons, and this particular Sunday was no exception. Strangely enough, the theme of his sermon was how many of us fail to recognize the Lord's presence in our everyday affairs. In the postman who smiles, the neighbor who visits us and offers a helping hand when we need it most. Yes, he even mentioned the motorist who stops to offer a helping hand."

"You've got to be kidding," said Tom from the back seat. "You really heard a sermon like that the next day?"

"Honest, Tom," replied my wife, "we did."

We had arrived at our friends' home and the hour was late. They were insisting that we come in, but we just couldn't and with some regrets they opened the back door to leave. Just before they left, Mary Alice asked me, "Joe, just one last question. Why were your knuckles only a mild blue instead of white?"

"Close the car door for a second and I'll tell you."

"Oh, what now," chuckled Tom.

"Well, it was like this. The night before the trip I was experiencing my usual early aerophobic symptoms. You know, butterflies, stomach acid, and such. Instead of reaching for a bromo, I reached for a book of Old Testament bible psalms on our bedside table. Picking up the book I flipped through the pages and, believe it or not, the first psalm my eyes fell on contained the sentence, 'The Lord will protect your journey and your homecoming.'"

"Oh my gosh!" replied Mary Alice, "How come you have such a direct line with the Lord? I never get any messages or answers like that!"

The snowfall was starting to taper off as the procession of cars reached the grave site. I recalled that I didn't answer her that night, but only laughed. What Mary Alice didn't realize was that she was part of the message, yes, part of God's message to any or all of us whose lives she had touched. She herself, radiating the simple trust of the small child, didn't need any messages. It was a poor stumbling, fearful child like myself that needed constant reassurances from our loving Father, who in His great generosity had to hit me on the head every now and then to remind me of His unfailing love and protection.

When I look back on her life and the ten odd years we knew her, her greatest gift to me, probably to all who knew her, was this trust she had in Divine Providence. Her death particularly exemplified this. Despite her intense suffering, she was the littlest of children in her total surrender and abandonment into the hands of her loving Father, God.

The mourners were clustered about the coffin bearing Mary Alice's remains. A green canopy was overhead and chairs were set up on a carpet spread under the canopy. The elderly and relatives were seated in the chairs. The priest read the final prayers in front of the coffin, which was bedecked with a beautiful arrangement of red carnations. After he finished, Tom and his daughters went forward and touched the coffin. Tom then started taking some of the carnations from atop the coffin and handed them to the mourners who came forward to offer one last word of sympathy to him and to his girls. We were two of the last to step forward. Jean and Tom hugged one another as he gave her a carnation. She then hugged his daughters. I then shook Tom's hand and offered my own condolences to him and the girls. We then slowly left the grave site and filed back to our cars. Getting inside the car, Jean and I sat in silence, waiting for the rest of the mourners to leave.

Looking at the red carnation that my wife was holding, I broke the silence. "Look at the petals, honey, just below the flower." Two large green petals were folded gracefully upward on the stem in the shape of a heart. The outline was unmistakable. Jean sadly smiled and then softly replied, "She was more than my best friend. She was closer than a sister to me."

The snow was now only a trickle as solitary flakes fell and stuck to the car window. So beautiful was the outline and pattern of each flake, so unique. Why couldn't they remain with us longer? Why did they have to melt so quickly?

Oh yes, I almost forgot, Mary Alice died in Mother Mary's arms, clothed in her Scapular of Carmel.

— 22 —

Little Things

At the present moment I am sitting in an airport in Miami with my son Joe. We are on our way to Kingston, Jamaica to work in Fr. Richard Albert's health clinics servicing the poorest of the poor. It should be a rewarding experience; I will care for the children and Joe for the adults. In addition to being a cancer specialist, he is a first-rate internist.

I can't believe it, but once again I have forgotten to do one of those "little things" for a friend of mine. You have plenty of time to think while traveling, and I just recalled the hernia belt I promised to send Fr. James some months ago. He is one of the missionaries I correspond with, and he wrote me some time ago, telling me that he had given away the belt I sent him three years ago. He gave it to a poor old man who needed it more than he did. I am feeling very guilty recalling the fact that our gracious Lord never forgets "little things." I promised myself to take care of it as soon as I return.

It was the summer before last, on a trip to Buffalo, New York to visit my mother, when our loving Saviour demonstrated to me in a unique manner not only the value of little things, but His infinite mercy and forgiveness as well.

It was the first week in July, and by happy coincidence another one of the missionary priests that I correspond with, Fr. Joseph Manapallil from Kerala, India was also planning a trip to the United States to visit a priest friend of his in Buffalo. Knowing this, I planned that we would get together and at the same time arrange to have him meet my mother and sister. One of his projects is improving housing for his very poor parishioners, and I wanted him to tell my family about it so perhaps they could organize some help for him.

Jean often makes the trip to Buffalo with me, but her new full-time nursing job as head allergy nurse at one of the local hospitals made it impossible this time. We would be celebrating our thirty-second wedding anniversary on my return, and I wanted to make sure I got a nice anniversary card for her. I spend a great deal of time when looking for an appropriate card, and of great concern to me is the verse. I want it to be just right and not a bit artificial.

The first day in Buffalo, after attending daily Mass with Mom and Ann Marie, my younger sister, we had breakfast together. It is always a festive occasion when we get together, sharing news about our respective families and most important of all, sharing our same ardent faith and talking about our mutual Loves, the Lord Jesus and His wonderful Mother Mary. They knew through previous correspondence that I planned to go to Fr. Manapallil's Mass the next morning at a parish some 20 miles from my sister's home, and that after Mass I would bring him back for a visit and brunch.

My mom, although she is now in her late eighties and has two artificial hips, is a pretty spry old gal and still manages to get around.

Sitting across from me as we finished breakfast she asked with an Irish grin, "What are you planning to do this morning, Joe?"

"I plan to look for an anniversary card for Jean, Mom; our anniversary is next week."

"The sixteenth of July, isn't it, Joe?" asked Ann Marie.

"Right; you have a good memory, Ann Marie. In fact, it's our thirty-second." Dabbing my mouth with a napkin I pulled back from the table and added, "In fact, you're going to have to excuse me because I must get going...you know how difficult it is picking out just the right card and verse."

Mom groaned and replied, "How well I do! You can spend the whole day trying to find the right one."

Ann Marie added with a laugh, "Sometimes it's better to write your own."

Smiling in agreement and heading for the door I replied, "Say some prayers to St. Anthony for me."

"St. Anthony, thank you," I thought to myself as with disbelief I found the perfect card in the first store I looked. Of all places, it was a drug store in the neighborhood where I grew up. The card had some attractive roses on the front, a genuine love note inside and a large white envelope in which to put it. When I came to the checkout counter to pay for the card I noticed some small, chocolate-covered peppermint patties which I have difficulty resisting. I purchased six of them with the silent resolve that I would eat only one and save the rest for Ann Marie and Mom.

I returned to the car, took out the card to admire it once more and then put it back in the white envelope. I placed it on the passenger seat and then decided to explore some of my home town haunts. I first drove by Christ the King Grammar School, where I had received the first eight years of my education. Looking at the window behind which was the original third grade, I recalled Sr. Consolata, my third grade teacher who had treated me so kindly. As a child I used to stutter, and she would very patiently wait while I, with difficulty, would struggle to get certain words out. Her kindness has never been forgotten. I then drove by the home where I spent most of my youth. I parked the car across the street and sat inside admiring the still, beautiful lawn that Dad had worked on so much — and had enlisted my reluctant help on so many occasions.

While enjoying these pleasant memories, I suddenly had the urge to sample one of the chocolate-covered peppermint patties. In no time at all I was smacking my lips as I devoured it. It was so good that I decided to try another...and then another; before I knew it, they were gone. "Ann Marie and Mom don't need the extra calories," I grunted to myself just before the guilt wave with its strong undertow hit me. While waiting for a traffic light to change, my eyes momentarily shifted to the passenger seat where during my orgy I had carelessly tossed the candy wrappers. In horror, I noticed that the white envelope was now covered with dark brown spots, caused by chocolate clinging to the wrappers which had inadvertently landed on the white envelope. Painfully looking at it, I visualized in my mind Sr. Consolata staring at me as she explained to we third graders the difference between mortal and venial sin.

"Children," she would say, "see the white bib I wear; well, if you commit venial sin, in the eyes of God your soul will become all spotted with dark spots, just like my bib would look if I splashed ink on it. If you commit a mortal sin, then your soul would be coal black and ugly, just as if I dunked this bib in a can of black paint."

"Oh, no!" I thought to myself as I imagined the envelope reflecting a picture of my soul at that moment while I wondered how I was going to get those spots off, or if unable to do so, where I was going to find another white envelope to replace the odd-sized one Jean's card was in.

Forgotten was the stained envelope as I attended Fr. Manapallil's Mass the next morning. I recall how impressed I was with the very devout manner in which he offered the Holy Sacrifice. Particularly so at the Consecration, when he slowly and deliberately pronounced the solemn words bringing Jesus to the altar and then reverently raised and lowered the Precious Body and Blood of our Lord and Saviour. After Mass we went over to the parish rectory and chatted a bit as he told me about the very poor area in which he served as pastor. "Although very poor, Dr. Evers, my parishioners are very devout. The church is always open and there are frequent Eucharistic visitors." I sighed and replied, "How different are things in America, Father. Many of our churches are locked up except when there are services. This is done because of fear of robbery and desecration. How lonely is our Saviour in the Eucharist in America." Silently and sadly he nodded his head in agreement with my remarks. We talked a bit longer and then left for the planned brunch.

Father, a small, slender man in his early fifties, enjoyed the morning with my mother and sister and the very tasty meal that had been prepared. He explained to all of us the shelters he was attempting to construct for his poor parishioners, and Mom and Ann Marie promised they would do their best to aid him. After lunch we said the Rosary together, but with a 20-mile drive ahead of us and with overcast skies threatening rain, we concluded the visit a little earlier than expected.

We hadn't been on the road more than ten minutes when it started to rain. It was a warm, gentle rain but looked at though it would last awhile. I was keeping to the speed limit, going about 40 miles an hour and talking with Father when suddenly at a major intersection I spied out of the corner of my eye a lady in rags standing on the curb begging alms. I felt the strongest urge to stop and give her a little money, but the light was green, it was raining and it seemed awkward if not dangerous to do so.

Some 15 minutes later we were at our destination and I left Father off. We mutually promised to resume our correspondence when we returned to our respective homes.

I started the 20-mile drive back, and it continued to rain. As I neared the intersection at which I had previously seen the lady beggar I was surprised to see her still there with her cup in her hand and a bag at her feet. The urge to help returned. I pulled the car into a nearby shopping mall and walked some hundred yards back to where she was standing. Fortunately, I had an umbrella and needed it as the rain was coming down harder than ever. Before I realized it I was just a few feet from her. She was a dark-skinned, middle-aged woman with a wrinkled face. She had a dirty red bandanna wrapped around her head and wore an oversized dark brown raincoat that looked very ragged and worn.

I went up to her, smiled, pulled out my wallet and reached inside, pulling out a $10 bill. In another section of my wallet I had a picture of Jesus crowned with thorns. I easily found it and instinctively wrapped the bill around the picture and gave it to her. "This is for you," I said. She did not reply. Without smiling she reached into the old duffel bag at her feet, pulled out a pencil and gave it to me. I thanked her for it and stuck it into my raincoat pocket and returned to the car.

Once inside the car I noticed that the pencil had a white eraser. I had kept the chocolate-spotted envelope on the passenger car seat, and without thinking I reached for it and started erasing the spots with the white eraser. I gasped, for it worked perfectly; within a few seconds the envelope was spotless. Reflecting on my gluttonous and selfish previous behavior, tears welled in my eyes, tears of thanksgiving at realizing how good God is, how filled with mercy and forgiveness. He used a little one disguised as a beggar and a little thing like a white eraser to so well demonstrate this to me that rainy afternoon.

While in Kingston, Jamaica working with my son Joe in Fr. Richard Alberts' health clinics, I observed more than once with parental pride as Joe did little things well. I recall him counseling a patient with high blood pressure as he counted out pills, placing them in a small envelope. Looking at the elderly man, I remember him saying in a voice mixed with concern and kindness, "Remember, these pills are not going to cure your disease, but they will control it provided that you replenish your supply when you run out. Just come back to the clinic and the nurse will give you more pills. It is more important for you to remember that you must take them every day for the rest of your life." He kept stressing this last point as he gently helped the man off the examining table and carefully guided him toward the door.

Last year Joe joined a large Oncology group in Richmond, Virginia where he now lives with his wife, Barbara, and their two small boys, Taylor and Ryan. Before they moved they were but a scant 30-minute drive away. Jean and I sure miss them, and I particularly miss four-year-old Taylor, our oldest grandson. When they lived near us I used to take Taylor, then three going on four, out with me on my days off. We did neat things like feed the ducks, go to the zoo, sing songs and throw rocks. One particular place he liked to go was to our local church. I would sit down in a pew with him on my lap (he is a very cuddly little boy) and sing hymns to him at the top of my voice. The church was almost always empty, so I was able to easily do this. His favorites were "Amazing Grace" and "Morning Has Broken." Occasionally the organist was there practicing, and she always smiled at us and gave a special little performance for Taylor.

We were in the habit of lighting two candles for his mom and dad before leaving the church, and I recall one day after his baby brother had been born that after we had lit the two candles he resisted leaving the niche where the candle rack was. I looked quizzically at him and he looked up at me with those blue eyes of his , and arching his eyebrows, he whispered in a barely audible voice, "Don't forget Ryan, Papa." Of course! I had forgotten his new baby brother. I then guided his little hand and let him light one more. After lighting the candles we knelt down and said a prayer. Before we left the church he would put his mouth to his lips and blow a kiss to baby Jesus in the tabernacle.

Well do I recall once on a dreary October afternoon as I was leaving the church hand in hand with him that I was prompted to say, "Taylor, do you know that God loves the prayers of little innocent children and they are among His favorites." He looked up at me with an understanding look on his face, waiting for me to continue. "Do you know that your prayer ascends like an arrow up to the highest heavens into the throne room of God, landing at His feet." With the sweetest smile on his face and still looking up at me he replied, "No, no Papa, it doesn't go up like an arrow, it goes up like a rocket!" I laughed as he said this and affirming his innocent insight, echoed, "You're right, Taylor, it goes up like a rocket."

There was a bench nearby and Taylor said, "Sit down, Papa." I didn't know what he had in mind but did as he requested. He then ran some 20 feet from me to where some green ferns were growing. Bending over a very small two-leafed one, he broke off one of the ferns. Cradling it in his hands, he carried it like a priceless treasure over to me. Stretching his hands out toward me he said very solemnly, "This is for you, Papa...I love you, Papa." I was emotionally overwhelmed for a moment by my dear little grandson and his magnanimous gift. It was a very "little thing" to all appearances, but in his eyes it was a precious gem that he was giving to his Papa. What made it precious was the love that it came wrapped in.

Reflecting on the incident later, I wonder if God, our loving Father, does not feel the same way when we His children, imitating the virtues so well captured by my little grandson, offer to Him each day many "little things" out of pure love. The Blessed Mother plays a very important role in this, for when living the life of "Spiritual Childhood" our daily thoughts, words and deeds — now motivated by love — are arranged by her like a bouquet of flowers and presented to God through her hands on our behalf.

Oh! I almost forgot. I did mail the hernia belt to Fr. John James, and three weeks later received the following reply: "Doctor Evers, thank you so much for the belt, the poor old beggar came to my door just a day or so after it arrived and I inquired how he was doing. He replied that all was going well except that his hernia belt was in shreds and did I have another. He is now wearing the belt you so kindly sent."

Guess what I must promptly do.

Biography

Dr. Evers and his wife Jean live in McLean Virginia where he has been in the private practice of Pediatrics for the past 37 years. A native of Buffalo, New York, Dr. Evers graduated from Canisius College in 1951 with a Bachelor of Science degree. Following his acceptance into Georgetown Medical School, he moved to Washington D.C. where he graduated with a medical degree in 1955. He continued his medical training with a rotating internship at D.C. General Hospital and then entered a three year Pediatric residency program starting with a one year program at Georgetown Hospital and finishing with a two year program at Children's Hospital (now Children's National Medical Center) Washington, D.C.

Upon completion of his Pediatric training he began pediatric solo practice in McLean, Virginia, a suburban community just outside Washington D.C. In 1964 he entered into a pediatric partnership with Dr. Enrico Davoli which continues to this day.

Dr. Evers is a charter member of the Alpha Omega Alpha Honor Medical Society at Georgetown Schooll of Medicine and at present serves as a Clinical Assistant Professor of Pediatrics on the staff of the Georgetown University School of Medicine. In 1992, he was invested as a Knight of Malta.